DATE DUE

2/29/00			
GAYLORD			PRINTED IN U.S.A.

ETHICAL AND LEGAL ISSUES
IN AIDS RESEARCH

ETHICAL AND LEGAL ISSUES IN AIDS RESEARCH

Joni N. Gray and Phillip M. Lyons, Jr.
Law/Psychology Program,
University of Nebraska, Lincoln

and

Gary B. Melton
Institute for Families in Society,
University of South Carolina, Columbia

The Johns Hopkins University Press • Baltimore and London

The Johns Hopkins University Press
2715 North Charles Street
Baltimore, Maryland 21218-4319
The Johns Hopkins Press Ltd., London

ISBN 0-8018-4910-1
ISBN 0-8018-4946-2 (pbk.)

Library of Congress Cataloging-in-Publication Data will be found
at the end of this book.
A catalog record for this book is available from the British Library.

CONTENTS

FOREWORD

The AIDS epidemic has taught us many lessons. Most of these lessons we could have done without, but some have been valuable. Like the canary sent into the mine, AIDS has tested the status of our science, our health care systems, and our ethics. This book outlines many of the ethical and research lessons for social and behavioral scientists that have resulted from the challenges posed by HIV/AIDS.

To understand our current situation, it may be helpful to think of three distinct epidemics, as often described by Jonathan Mann (1988). The first epidemic is of the human immunodeficiency virus (HIV), the virus that causes AIDS. Although the virus has likely been around for many decades in one form or another, it took hold in an epidemic sense in the United States in the middle to late 1970s. As Walter Cronkite was describing the Bicentennial in 1976, no one was aware that the most significant epidemic of modern times was spreading silently among clusters of people in cities that later would become epicenters. The Tall Ships in New York Harbor and the San Francisco fireworks were part of that Bicentennial celebration. In both cities, the HIV epidemic had already taken hold.

The second epidemic is of AIDS itself, the mysterious syndrome that develops following infection with HIV. It was first reported in July 1981 and appeared to affect only young gay men. Was it due to excessive stress on the immune system from living in the fast lane? Or was it a new sexually transmitted disease? By 1983, everyone in the gay community had an opinion; those who believed in the blood-borne virus theory even began a controversial campaign for safer sexual practices. By March 1985, the virus had been identified, and a biological marker, an antibody test, was available. We then moved into the age of the "infected" and the "uninfected."

The public policy and ethical issues associated with the availability of a biological marker have continued ever since.

The third epidemic can be characterized as the social, economic, and political reactions in the wake of the HIV and AIDS epidemics. Because the HIV and AIDS epidemics have enormous consequences in terms of resources and resource allocation, they must be viewed in the larger context of their impact on societies, cultures, countries, and the globe. In parts of Africa, the young workers necessary for agricultural development are gone, thus changing the future of whole regions of the continent. In the United States, the number of years of life lost before age sixty-four because of AIDS now surpasses those lost to both cancer and heart disease. The major economic impact of the epidemics is just beginning. In 1994, the U.S. government will provide more than $6 billion for disability, medical, and public health programs. This epidemic costs more than any natural disaster we have experienced to date, and it continues to grow each year. As epidemic-related costs continue to stretch the federal budget, the debate over the allocation of resources will become more bitter.

As a gay man living in San Francisco, one of the epicenters of the HIV and AIDS epidemics, I have experienced the impact of AIDS very personally. By the summer of 1993, more than 11,000 gay men had died of AIDS in San Francisco, and more than 28,000 were living with HIV infection. Despite extensive prevention campaigns, more than 600 new infections among gay men are projected in the city each year. Nearly half of all gay men in San Francisco are infected. AIDS has claimed my primary care physician, my dermatologist, my last two dentists, three hair cutters, and even my mail carrier. Of more than 300 people who attended a fundraiser I hosted in the early 1980s, over one-third are now dead. Last year, I lost my best friend. For me, AIDS is primarily a personal issue.

As a psychologist, I have been impressed with the importance of understanding human behavior in any attempts to respond to the AIDS crisis. Because HIV generally is transmitted by voluntary behaviors, either sexual or drug-sharing, the interruption of transmission must be based on an understanding of these behaviors. Risk reduction requires changing individual behavior and community norms. Thus, behavior research on HIV prevention is of critical importance in controlling the spread of the virus.

Many of the important policy issues debated by the American Psychological Association's Task Force on Psychology and AIDS, which I chaired, and the later Ad Hoc Committee on Psychology and AIDS, are outlined in detail in this book. Like the larger society, the scientific and helping professions have been stressed by this crisis. Perhaps this is most obvious in the discussions of HIV and the duty to protect. My experience, over and over again, has been that very well-qualified clinicians lose their clinical skills when working with an HIV-infected client/patient. Unfortunately, however, attempts to give guidance to clinicians on how to handle these situations have been blocked repeatedly by well-meaning provider representatives fearful of giving the wrong advice. The breakdown of normal decision making is a predictable part of the third epidemic of social and political disruption in the wake of the virus and disease.

As one deeply involved in public policy, I have learned that AIDS is always political. Issues like needle exchange, adolescent sex surveys, travel restrictions, requirements to inform research participants of their serostatus, restrictions on the content of prevention materials, objections to the marketing of condoms, restrictions that material not in any way promote the acceptance of homosexuality, and so forth, are all part of the political context of the HIV and AIDS epidemics. Clearly, fear blocks thoughtful and humane responses to this crisis. Bad public policy in turn interferes with shaping an adequate response to the HIV and AIDS epidemics.

The authors of this book are to be commended for presenting objective data and findings that are behind the scientific and public policy debates. An understanding of the ethical and legal issues in AIDS research yields insights into the answers to the major challenges of responding to the broader AIDS crisis.

Steve Morin, Ph.D.
Office of Congresswoman Nancy Pelosi
U.S. House of Representatives

PREFACE

The idea for this book arose during the mid-1980s, when one of us (Gary Melton) chaired the American Psychological Association (APA) Committee for the Protection of Human Participants in Research (CPHPR, later known as the Committee on Standards in Research). During that time two of us served on APA AIDS task forces: the APA Task Force on Psychology and AIDS (the forerunner to the standing Committee on Psychology and AIDS) (Gary Melton) and the APA Division 37 Task Force on Pediatric AIDS (Joni Gray). In those early days of the AIDS epidemic, virtually every issue that CPHPR considered seemed to emanate from problems in the design and conduct of research on AIDS.

A sample of the issues that CPHPR considered illustrates the range of thorny problems that arise when researchers study problems related to AIDS:

— Is mandatory participation in research ever ethically permissible?
— Should participants in research be required to learn personally relevant information?
— Do the ethics of research change when the topic is socially sensitive?
— Under what circumstances, if ever, is it permissible to seek research involvement of individuals who are in public places (e.g., bathhouses, gay bars) but engaged in what they probably would regard as private behavior?
— Should researchers be required to consult with the community of potential participants about the ethics of their research?
— Should the protection offered by federal confidentiality certificates (see Melton, 1990) be broadened?
— When should identifiable research data be made available to third par-

ties (whether private parties or public health authorities) without the participants' consent?
— Is clinical competence a requisite for research on personally sensitive matters?
— Is political or cultural competence a requisite for socially sensitive research? (Melton, 1991a, p. 561)[1]

Two general conclusions that are relevant to the scope of this book can be drawn from this list. First, the issues identified were not specific to AIDS, but the complexity of interests involved in AIDS research and the life-or-death seriousness of the resolution of such conflicts of interest sharpened the ethical issues that are involved more generally in research involving human participants. Consequently, a number of the revisions of the Ethical Principles of Psychologists (APA, 1992)—and numerous other proposed revisions that ultimately were not accepted—were generated as a direct result of the CPHPR discussions about AIDS research, even though the new provisions were obviously not limited to that content area.

Similarly, although this volume is focused on AIDS research, much of the information and analysis it contains is germane to research involving human participants in general. Readers will note parallels to work in other socially and personally sensitive domains, particularly within the public health field. In that sense, although the field of AIDS research has grown at an extraordinary rate, much of the discussion in this volume is likely to have usefulness in a broader range of contexts for a longer period of time than may be typical for reviews of other topics in the field. (Readers should be aware, of course, that the law may change—as frequently occurs because of the adoption of special statutes on matters pertaining to AIDS—and that they should consult counsel about the law prevailing in their own state in particular situations.)

Second, although the greater emphasis in this book is on *psychosocial* research related to AIDS, most of the discussion is also relevant to human *biomedical* research on AIDS. Most of the issues that CPHPR considered could have arisen as easily in an analogous committee of a medical research society. Our emphasis on psychosocial research is a product in part of our own background in psychology and law and, as a result, of our greater familiarity with examples from the social and behavioral sciences. Also,

---

1. The issues were sufficiently diverse and complex that Melton drafted a set of guidelines for research on AIDS that were adopted by CPHPR (1982, 1985) in consultation with the APA Committee on Lesbian and Gay Concerns.

the Ethical Principles of Psychologists (APA, 1992) comprise the most comprehensive professional code for ethical conduct in human research. Psychological research pertaining to AIDS thus offers a convenient area for the analysis of ethical norms as they prevail in the scientific community.

The focus is not just for expedience, however. Some of the most complex and controversial ethical problems in AIDS research have arisen in the context of the study of behavior. For example, how can the risk of HIV infection associated with particular behavior that is illegal or private be discovered without undue intrusion on privacy? Similarly, many of the thorniest problems in biomedical research on AIDS have been dependent at least in part on assumptions about the emotional or behavioral consequences of biomedical research. For example, research policy decisions have been based on assumptions about (a) the consequences of unrequested disclosures to participants of the results of HIV-antibody tests that they took as part of a research protocol, and (b) the psychological effects of participation in clinical trials using placebo controls.

Although we will discuss and argue about overarching ethical issues, nuts-and-bolts legal issues also require attention. Consequently, readers will note two broad levels of analysis and discussion in this book. The book begins and ends with a consideration of overarching ethical problems, the dilemmas that permeate research on AIDS, and a presentation of arguments about the interests that should be paramount. At the same time, however, the resolution of these grand dilemmas is contingent on an understanding of the nuts and bolts of the law. Therefore, we necessarily focus much of the book on technical problems of law, as they are applied to research on AIDS. Chapters 2 through 5 address these technical matters in some detail and provide insight into how courts and other legal decision makers resolve them. Although our discussion addresses these legal issues with some specificity, our treatment of these topics should be read in the light of the more global ethical considerations that precede and introduce the technical legal chapters.

Our ideas about the ethical issues involved in AIDS research were stimulated in part during the CPHPR discussions. As colleagues on CPHPR, Michael Saks, Joan Sieber, and Barbara Stanley were collaborators in a series of projects to illuminate ethical problems in psychological research, and their ideas and questions have influenced our analyses.

Stimulating discussions were also provided by a working group commissioned by CPHPR to study psychological questions that arose in the initial trials of drugs for the treatment of AIDS and the ethical and political discussions thereafter. In addition to Melton, members of the working group included Gerald Koocher, Robert Levine, Robert Rosenthal, and William Thompson. Melton was also fortunate to participate in another APA working group that analyzed ethical problems in psychological research related to homosexuality (see Herek, Kimmel, Amaro & Melton, 1991).

Acknowledgment is also due to the staff of the Center on Children, Families, and the Law who assisted with library research. Rene Williams was particularly helpful with last-minute work in that regard.

Much of our discussion of AIDS research issues pertaining to children was influenced by Joni Gray's participation on the APA Task Force on Pediatric AIDS. This group produced a report on a broad range of issues pertaining to children, adolescents, and AIDS (Seibert & Olson, 1989; see also Gray, 1989 for more specific coverage of pediatric AIDS research issues). Many of the ideas presented in this book have appeared in earlier works by the authors on the law and ethics of AIDS research (Gray, 1989; Gray & Melton, 1985; Henggeler, Melton & Rodrigue, 1992, Chap. 7; Melton, 1988, 1989, 1991a, 1991b; Melton & Gray, 1988; Melton et al., 1988).

ETHICAL AND LEGAL ISSUES IN AIDS RESEARCH

Chapter 1

THE INTERESTS AT STAKE

"We are the first, so we try to keep this," said [Luc] Montagnier, speaking of scientific reputation as though it were a tennis ranking. "Now there are many competitors. It is more difficult to be at the top of the research. We are trying to be the first for a vaccine, for therapeutics, for improving diagnostic technique."

If Montagnier ever was shy and retiring, he is no longer. In a recent discussion of his work, the 55-year-old scientist came across as ambitious, competitive and proud. And to Montagnier, the scientist, confronting the AIDS crisis has brought the most fascinating and stimulating research he has ever directed—coupled with the chance to travel the world, influencing scientific and political leaders.

R. Herman, "Pasteur's Leader in AIDS Research"

Defining the Issues

Two or three years after acquired immunodeficiency syndrome (AIDS) was first identified (Centers for Disease Control, 1981; Gottleib et al., 1981), researchers in Bethesda (Robert Gallo), Paris (Luc Montagnier), and San Francisco (Jay Levy) nearly simultaneously and seemingly independently isolated the virus that caused the mysterious and deadly disease (e.g., Barre-Sinoussi et al., 1983; Gallo et al., 1984). The social significance of the discovery was obvious. It provided the basis for the rapid development of a test that would detect antibodies to the virus and thus provide a means for screening blood donations for exposure to it. The safety of blood transfusions could be assured again. The breakthrough also opened the door to research for treatments and vaccines that would attack the cause of AIDS. A major step had been taken down the long road toward the control of the AIDS epidemic.

The discovery of the virus causing AIDS would surely bring world acclaim to the researchers involved—perhaps a Nobel prize. Nearly immediately, the patent resulting from the development of the test for antibodies to the virus would bring substantial income to the researchers' sponsor.

There was also substantial political benefit for governments beleaguered by protests of purported slothfulness in responding to the AIDS crisis—a fact that did not go unnoticed by the U.S. Secretary of Health and Human Services, who scheduled a high-profile press conference to announce the findings of Gallo and his colleagues at the National Cancer Institute.

Another nearly immediate result was a dispute between Gallo and Montagnier about who deserved the credit (Norman, 1985). International litigation (*Institut Pasteur v. United States*, 1987) ensued to determine the validity of the patent for the antibody test. Settlement came only after shuttle diplomacy by Jonas Salk and a White House ceremony at which Presidents Reagan and Chirac signed an agreement recognizing Gallo and Montagnier as "co-discoverers" (Shilts, 1987).

Meanwhile, an international committee of retrovirus researchers was convened to seek a solution to what the chair described as the "intractably confusing and at times overly contentious issue" (Varmus, 1989, p. 3) of the name for the virus. Was it human T-lymphotrophic virus type III (HTLV-III, as Gallo had named it), lymphadenopathy-associated virus (LAV, as Montagnier had christened it), AIDS-related virus (ARV, as Levy had termed it), or, diplomatically, HTLV-III/LAV or HTLV-III/LAV/ARV? The compromise choice of most members of the committee was human immunodeficiency virus (HIV), although Gallo refused to join Levy and Montagnier in signing the letters to the editors of *Nature* and *Science* that announced the decision in May 1986.

The dispute has continued with allegations of (a) misrepresentation of the data by Gallo or others in his lab, (b) misappropriation of the Pasteur Institute virus by Gallo, and (c) ineptitude and unfairness in the resulting investigation by the Office of Research Integrity of the National Institutes of Health (NIH)—an early test of the diligence of NIH in responding to allegations of scientific fraud (Hamilton, 1991; Palca, 1991; Rubinstein, 1991). The dispute has further pitted influential members of Congress against NIH, and it has provided an avenue for political squabbles between branches of the Public Health Service (PHS).

On November 13, 1993, the Office of Research Integrity dropped its charges of ethical misconduct against Gallo. The Office stated that its actions were the result of the application by the Department of Health and Human Services' appeals board of "different standards from those applied by the Office of Research Integrity" (Hilts, 1993). Despite the office's statement that the dismissal was based on changes in evidentiary standards, Gallo, perhaps unsurprisingly, announced that he "ha[d] been completely vindicated" (Hilts, 1993). The battle, however, is not over. Undaunted, lawyers for the Pasteur Institute reaffirmed its commitment to pursuit of more credit for the French (Hilts, 1993).

Using People for the Good of Society—and of Researchers

The narcissism and competition for profits that have been displayed in the continuing saga of the discovery of HIV seem better suited for a story-line in a Tom Clancy or John Grisham novel than in the pages of *Science*. By starting with it, we do not mean to imply that scientific integrity is the core ethical issue in research on AIDS. Rather, we describe the Gallo-Montagnier feud to illustrate a point that is seldom given due emphasis in discussions of research ethics: researchers have substantial conflicts of interest. Scientific research involves the *use* of people for society's good—and the researcher's tenure, promotion, merit pay, and public and collegial admiration. When (as is obviously the case in AIDS research) the public interest in the acquisition of knowledge is great, so too is the researcher's property interest. Ironically, therefore, the more important that research is to society, the greater is the potential for researchers to have conflicts of interest. Although most research does not carry the same stakes or extraordinary significance as the discovery of HIV, the example is nevertheless instructive.

In recognizing that point, one need not—and should not—attribute a nefarious or avaricious motive to researchers involved in socially important studies. Intellectual property law is based on the assumption that rewards for individual creativity will result in a greater production of knowledge and, ultimately, greater enhancement of social welfare.[1] The scientific enterprise thus is structured to provide incentives, prestige and money, for useful innovations. Moreover, a primary focus on pecuniary rewards probably would have led researchers to other occupational choices. Researchers in the social and health sciences make a commitment to use their education and intellect for altruistic purposes. Because researchers' pursuit of their own welfare often has benefit for social welfare and because researchers typically are also motivated to promote social good, conflicts of interest are rarely clear.

Researchers are not the only parties with mixed motives, though. So-

---

1. This assumption also colors other areas of law in which action that might interrupt the scientific enterprise is at issue (see, e.g., *Andrews v. Eli Lilly & Co.*, 1983; *Dow Chemical Co. v. Allen*, 1982; *Richards of Rockford v. Pacific Gas & Electric*, 1976).

ciety itself may be concerned with improving the welfare of research participants and others like them, but it may also be interested in using knowledge derived from research to control the populations from which participants are selected. If the latter motive is strong enough, it may even justify compulsory "participation" in research.[2]

Participants, too, may have mixed interests. Participants may have purely altruistic motives, or they may cope with a seemingly senseless situation by contributing to knowledge about it and thus giving it some meaning and themselves some satisfaction and solace. Participants or others like them with whom they identify may also be perceived as potentially directly benefiting from the research. Even if the probability of personal benefit is remote, it may be accepted with some desperation by people with life-threatening diseases, who may be willing to tolerate considerable discomfort and inconvenience in the service of science.

Conflicts of Interest in Public Health

Few situations present the dilemmas involved in conflicts of interest within and between groups more starkly than research on topics in public health.[3] On the one hand, inquiry about matters related to health clearly intrudes on privacy. Control over knowledge about oneself and particularly about one's body is necessary to ensure respect for persons and often constitutionally protected (Melton, 1983; *Merriken v. Cressman*, 1973; Ruebhausen & Brim, 1966; *United States v. Westinghouse Electric Corp.*, 1980; *Whalen v. Roe*, 1977). Loss of control over such information, whether through compelled disclosure or breach of confidentiality, subjects individuals to embarrassment and degradation (*Lora v. Board of Education*, 1977).

On the other hand, research related to public health has obvious benefit to society. Accordingly, it is well established in law that the state may ex-

---

2. The more traditional term, research *subjects*, connotes that the individuals involved in the production of data are in fact serving society, the researcher, or both, that is, that they are being used. We prefer to label such individuals *participants* to connote a partnership in which the researcher joins with others to increase knowledge. We also recognize, however, that when involvement is coerced, *participant* is simply a euphemism that obscures the actual power differential. We suspect, for example, that the description of introductory psychology students as *subjects* in research is a more accurate characterization of their experience. The same experience may apply to some clinical research that is not for participants' own benefit, in which informed consent is treated as a bureaucratic ritual rather than the establishment of a partnership (cf. Lidz et al., 1984).

3. This section is taken with minor revision from Melton and Gray (1988).

ercise the police power to curb threats to public health. As the Supreme Court noted in a landmark case shortly after the turn of the century, "There are manifold restraints to which every person is necessarily subject for the common good. On any other basis organized society could not exist with safety to its members. . . . Upon the principle of self-defense, of paramount necessity, a community has the right to protect itself against an epidemic of disease which threatens the safety of its members" (*Jacobson v. Massachusetts*, 1905, pp. 26–27).

That authority could be used to compel the production of information if, for example, behavioral-epidemiological or social network data were necessary to determine potential causes and paths of transmission of a disease. Case-cluster methods, such as those used to begin to determine the means of transmission of AIDS soon after it was discovered (Auerbach, Darrow, Jaffe & Curran, 1984; Centers for Disease Control, 1982; Klovdahl, 1985), border on state-compelled participation in research. Although participation in interviews by Auerbach et al. was consensual, contact of participants by governmental authorities occurred without their prior consent, and the story that was ultimately uncovered was reported in the popular press (Shilts, 1987).

Thus, when research relates to public health, conflicts may arise between respect for persons (and their privacy) and beneficence (the promotion of human welfare). This clash of principles ("The Belmont Report," 1979) is complicated further because participants in research related to public health may be especially vulnerable to harm flowing from intrusions on privacy. Beyond the abstract violation of a zone of privacy and the resulting threat to personal dignity, participants may be in danger of substantial direct harm. Questioning about one's status as a patient with a grave illness—or even the possibility of one's becoming a patient—is likely to engender distress. Moreover, disclosure of participants' status, even if simply as members of a risk group, may result in their being subjected to social stigma and legal sanctions (e.g., quarantine; punishment for engaging in prohibited risky behavior). Thus, prospective participants may have a clear interest in avoiding participation and, if they choose to participate, in preventing the disclosure of data to third parties.

At the same time, participants, particularly if they are patients themselves or at risk of becoming ill, have a profound interest in the promotion of research on the illness in question. They even have an interest in the retention of identifiable information when it might be used for longitudinal research, for sharing of data sets crucial to an understanding of the disease, or for the notification of individuals who may benefit from innovative treatments.

Conflicts of Interests in AIDS Research

AIDS presents especially stark and troubling examples of the ethical and legal problems in public health research. In part, the acuity of ethical issues in AIDS research is a product simply of the magnitude of the stakes— life or death for millions of people (and sometimes for individual research participants) around the world who already are infected with HIV.

The stakes also are high, though, because the participants may be risking the loss of their privacy and even their freedom. The cost of both participating and not participating can be enormous. Those whose time is used, whose lives are intruded upon, and whose bodies serve as objects of experimentation often are people who already are subject to discrimination and even criminal punishment, who are hidden because of stigma, and who are poor and vulnerable:

> AIDS . . . is an inhumane disease. Its virus fastens almost unerringly on humans already affected by special social and physical vulnerability. It attacks the fetus, whose ability to defend itself is almost nonexistent. It attacks women in poverty, who are often the coerced sexual partners of infected drug users. It invades the bodies of the drug addicted, whose will to resist has already been captured by their habit. It massacres the population of male homosexuals, whose freedoms are already threatened by prejudice. AIDS seems to seek out as its victims the weakest and the already victimized. . . . It is prejudiced, utterly destructive, and coldly cruel in its killing. (Jonsen, 1989, p. xi)

And, one might add, AIDS threatens the lives of people in much of the Third World and endangers the security of postcolonial societies that are just beginning to taste democracy and a decent standard of living—societies that still are dependent on in large part (or at least indebted to) the wealthy nations of the North, the nations from which most researchers come.

In such circumstances, the conflicts inherent in human research become particularly profound because of the powerlessness that people who may be "subjected" to research already experience. Their use by researchers on behalf of society in such a context makes the possibilities of harm to, or exploitation of, participants especially worrisome (e.g., Novick, 1990a).

Although *behavior*, not group membership, puts people at risk for HIV infection, the epidemiological patterns have been important in identifying the mode of transmission, natural history, and directions for the prevention of the disease. Additionally, the need for the development of effective prevention and treatment has been greatest in high-prevalence communities. Given the nature of the groups initially identified by the Centers for Disease Control (CDC) as being at high risk (i.e., gay men, intravenous drug users and their sexual partners, and, for several years, people of Haitian origin; see Centers for Disease Control, 1985b) and the stigma that is associated with HIV infection itself (Herek & Glunt, 1988), the mere identification as a participant in research on AIDS may result in harm, especially if confidentiality is breached. Simply locating potential participants may be intrusive and harmful.

The risk is magnified because research on AIDS, especially psychosocial research, inherently carries the researcher (and the participants) into highly personal, sensitive topic areas. Full understanding of the mode of transmission and evaluation of the effectiveness of preventive programs have required the gathering of data from people with HIV infection and comparison groups (including people at high risk of infection) about their sexual practices, drug use, medical history, personality, and travel, and about their acquaintances, friends, and lovers. Disclosure ("confession") of information about illicit drug use and sexual behavior may not only place one at risk of criminal penalties but also raise the specter of civil commitment (e.g., if behavior posing a danger to self or others is at issue), civil child protection proceedings, administrative sanctions (e.g., loss of public employment), or private discrimination.

History suggests that such fears are not altogether unjustified. Historically, race and public health measures have been associated in the same way that race and other draconian "self-defense" measures have been intertwined (Price, 1989b, discussing *Jew Ho v. Williamson*, 1890, and *Korematsu v. United States*, 1944). Analogizing to the Tuskegee syphilis experiment, many African Americans view AIDS as part of a conspiracy for genocide (Thomas & Quinn, 1991), and racial politics has dominated particular AIDS research projects (see, e.g., Anderson, 1991, on the debate in New York City on the initiation of needle-exchange pilot projects).

On the other side, though, just as the risks associated with research participation may rest disproportionately on people already vulnerable, they may obtain fewer benefits of research. In the AIDS epidemic, the *exclusion* of groups from research has raised as many questions of injustice.

Until Rock Hudson's death became national news and concerns about AIDS cases arose among heterosexuals, the press response to AIDS (initially identified as gay-related immune deficiency [GRID])—and the corresponding response of research policymakers—was tepid in comparison with the reaction to toxic shock syndrome and Legionnaires' disease. As one journalist summarized, "Editors were killing pieces, reporters told Curran [a CDC official], because they didn't want stories about gays and all those distasteful sexual habits littering their newspapers" (Shilts, 1987, p. 110).

Although the "gay plague" initially failed to evoke great concern in the Washington research establishment, the history of AIDS research since the political mobilization of the gay community has been that the lower the status of the affected population, the less attention it has received in research and the later the research has begun. More men have been enrolled in research than women, more gay men than intravenous drug users, more gay men in communities where they have political clout than gay men in communities without strong gay organizations, more adults than children and youth, more adolescents with hemophilia than adolescents with more "blameworthy" routes of transmission, more Americans than Africans and Asians, and so on.

To some degree, this phenomenon is the understandable result of the desire to do research quickly, with relatively easy recruitment of participants, relatively easy achievement of compliance with protocols, and relatively few confounding variables. Insofar as it is the product of simple avoidance of less "desirable" populations, however, the process is sheer prejudice and the result is pernicious. Although this maldistribution of AIDS research has received greatest attention with regard to drug trials (see, e.g., Hein, 1991; Levine, 1991; Nolan, 1990; Valleroy, 1990),[4] the scope of the problem is broader. For example, the lower in status a particular population is, the less is known about its customs as they may relate to the design of prevention programs.[5]

---

4. In Henggeler, Melton & Rodrigue (1992, pp. 117–119), we discussed the problems associated with access by children and youth to clinical trials. Such trials remain controversial, as do experiments in treatment of pregnant women. The study of the effects of zidovudine (AZT) on HIV-infected pregnant women was the first where the administration of a potentially toxic substance during pregnancy has been approved ("NIH Agency Begins Study," 1991). ACT UP, a militant advocacy group for people with AIDS, objected vociferously because of the side effects of the drug and the absence of HIV infection in the majority of children born to HIV-infected women.

5. The scope of psychosocial research relevant to AIDS is broad. *Behavioral-epidemiological*

The Current Context

Although society is far from controlling the AIDS epidemic, even within the United States (Brandt, 1988), knowledge about AIDS has grown at an extraordinary rate. Research on the disease now often dominates the *Journal of the American Medical Association,* the *New England Journal of Medicine,* the *American Journal of Public Health,* and *Science,* as well as several specialized journals.

The first decade of the AIDS epidemic also stimulated hundreds of legal cases, including about 200 criminal prosecutions (Sherman, 1991; for a list of such cases, see Gostin, 1990a, 1990b). Ethical norms related to

---

research has been important in the identification initially of modes of transmission of HIV and, more recently, of social-contextual variables in risky behavior (e.g., Schoenbaum et al., 1989, identifying social factors accounting for variations in the rates of HIV infection among intravenous drug users of various ethnicity)—information that is germane to the design of prevention programs.

Neuropsychological research is significant, because HIV crosses the blood-brain barrier early in infection, so dementia is the presenting symptom leading to a diagnosis of AIDS in about one-fourth of the cases (Bridge, 1988b; Navia, Jordan & Price, 1986). Because of its importance in the pathology of AIDS (Bridge, 1988a), neuropathology is a useful marker in evaluating the efficacy of treatment. Study of neuropsychological factors is also relevant to policy development, because of questions (for example, in consenting to research) about the competence of patients with AIDS.

Biobehavioral research is also important in another context. *Neuropsychoimmunological* research examines questions about the significance of psychological variables as cofactors in the causation of HIV infection and its progression. Such work examines the relation of stress to immune system functioning (for reviews, see Glaser & Kiecolt-Glaser, 1988; Kiecolt-Glaser & Glaser, 1988; for an example of such work, see Cohen, 1988).

Of course, research on risk perception and risk taking underlies much of the effort to design AIDS prevention programs. That work includes an examination of the significance of cofactors (e.g., substance abuse) in risk taking. Psychosocial research is also important in treatment research, with regard to the design of trials that will be accepted (in essence, the mental health aspects of medical interventions, especially experimental interventions) and the assessment and treatment of secondary mental health consequences of AIDS and HIV infection.

Policy and service design and administration are informed by research on the social context of AIDS—public attitudes, prejudice, and discrimination and the functioning of the various systems, including health care, involved in response to the epidemic. In all areas, given the epidemiology of AIDS, cultural factors must be considered. In that regard, within-group variation requires specific study. For example, there are huge variations among Hispanic groups in the United States in the prevalence, gender distribution, and mode of transmission of HIV infection (Diaz, Buehler, Castro & Ward, 1993).

For thoughtful analyses of the agenda for psychosocial research on AIDS, see the National Research Council reports on the topic (Miller, Turner & Moses, 1990; Turner, Miller & Moses, 1989).

AIDS continue to evolve. Questions regarding the acceptable uses of human participants and of the imperative for the generation of knowledge relevant to public health are likely to become even more complex as preventive measures (e.g., vaccine trials) become more widespread and risky.

More generally, issues in AIDS research may portend broader questions of the legitimate use of state authority to protect public health. Dean Monroe Price (1989a, 1989b), of the Cardozo Law School at Yeshiva University, argued that AIDS may reorder the relation between the individual and the state.[6] He even suggested that the need to provide AIDS education "suddenly to open windows into the minds and souls of millions . . . [may] be seen by powerful institutions as a moment for reshaping the American character in its totality, not just as a chance to adjust that character to the needs of the moment" (Price, 1989a, p. 16). In such a context, questioning the use of individuals for social good—and their own good—assumes ever greater significance.

Some Ethical and Legal Problems

As we begin our discussion of substantive legal matters, a preliminary observation is in order; there is little in the way of bodies of "AIDS research law" that informs decisions regarding the conduct of research involving people with HIV infection or AIDS. For example, in Chapter 5 we describe some of the issues surrounding the recognition of a researcher-subject privilege. That discussion borrows, as it must, from the body of law relating to the reporter's privilege.

Similarly, in Chapter 4 we address researchers' duty to protect third parties from harm resulting from HIV infection. Our analysis necessarily relies heavily on the duty to protect individuals from assaultive behavior. This is so because assaultive conduct has traditionally been at the core of the duty. Thus, as we present the legal contours of AIDS research we will discuss other areas of substantive law. As some of our discussion will make clear, even when legislatures have enacted statutes addressing confidentiality, access to records, or other issues, significant gaps often exist with regard to the meaning of those statutes, and it is up

6. A similar argument was made previously in regard to youth policy specifically (Melton, 1989). The desire to constrain adolescents' risky behavior may result in either greater intrusion on their privacy and liberty (i.e., heightened state intrusiveness and control) or greater recognition of privacy and liberty by facilitating access to drug treatment, condoms, and other services and products that may diminish risk.

to courts to fill those gaps. Thus, although our meandrous journey through other bodies of substantive law may seem tangential, it is in fact precisely the kind of exploration that courts will undergo when considering these matters.

Intrusiveness

At the core of many of the ethical issues in AIDS research, especially psychosocial research, are concerns about the limits of privacy. Given the social consequences of HIV infection and the risks to public health that are at stake, how much control should participants be able to exercise over personal information?

Consistent with the general principle to "accord appropriate respect to the fundamental rights, dignity, and worth of all people," the Ethical Principles of Psychologists (American Psychological Association [APA], 1992) expressly recognize broad duties to protect privacy, although psychologists are enjoined at the same time to remain "mindful that legal and other obligations may lead to inconsistency and conflict with the exercise of these rights" (Principle [Prin.] D). The Principles are particularly detailed in their discussion of the duty to maintain confidentiality (Standards [Stds.] 5, 6.16, & 6.25), but they also establish a duty to avoid undue intrusiveness in research (Stds. 5.03 & 6.17) and in general to avoid harming participants (Std. 1.14 & Prin. E).

Although discrimination on the ground of HIV seropositivity—or even suspicion that an individual is HIV-seropositive—is now illegal in many circumstances[7] (Americans with Disabilities Act, 1990 [see esp. § 12102(2), defining a disability]; *School Board v. Arline*, 1987), disclosure of test results may still result in direct harm to relationships. Moreover, breaches of confidentiality about sexual and drug-taking histories may subject participants to other direct harm, including civil and criminal penalties, social ostracism, and embarrassment. Even if direct *harm* does not occur, loss of control over such personal information *wrongs* participants, because it is a violation of their dignity. Given both the centrality of confidentiality concerns in debates about the ethics of AIDS research and the

7. However, some conduct that clearly discriminates against people with HIV infection or AIDS is still permissible. Two different courts recently concluded, for example, that employers providing benefits under programs within the purview of the Employee Retirement Income Security Act of 1974 may lower health benefit caps for AIDS-related treatment—even after the employees have begun to file claims (*McGann v. H. & H. Music Co.*, 1991; *Owens v. Storehouse*, 1993).

complexity of the legal provisions involved, much of this book (Chaps. 3–5) is devoted to issues related to confidentiality.

Other concerns about privacy also are important, however. Notably, most AIDS research raises questions about the limits of justifiable *intrusions* on privacy. As has been clear since the first case-cluster studies tracing links among gay men with AIDS and their sexual partners, such issues begin even with the recruitment of participants. Because risky behavior involves domains of life that nearly everyone regards as private and because individuals at high risk are most often in stigmatized groups, both the behavior itself and the people who engage in it are frequently hidden. Researchers interested in studying bathhouse users, prostitutes, and intravenous (IV) drug users cannot simply contact organizations to locate them.

Accordingly, researchers identifying potential participants may seem to be more like private detectives than scientists. The higher the risk is in a particular population and, therefore, the greater the interest of the group for AIDS researchers, the more likely that it is to be so far outside the mainstream that locating participants requires investigative procedures. For example, the recruitment of male transvestite prostitutes in Atlanta (Elifson et al., 1993), a group that ultimately was shown to have an extraordinarily high rate of HIV-seropositivity (68%), required both social mapping (observation to determine specific locations frequented by transvestite prostitutes) and snowball sampling (interviewing of prostitutes to identify other potential participants).

To the degree that the behavior of interest is public, its interruption and its observation (even if unnoticed) are intrusive. Patrons and employees of brothels do not expect to be approached by research assistants with questionnaires, interview protocols, and blood-test kits in hand (see, e.g., Khabbaz et al., 1990)![8]

Once a sample is recruited, the content of questionnaires or interviews is likely to infringe privacy. Detailed interviews about a participant's sexual practices and the number, identity, and sexual practices and preferences of the participant's sexual partners are not ordinary events. Although the

8. For other examples, see Elifson, Boles & Sweat (1993; study of male prostitutes on the street); Green, Goldberg, Nathwani, Christie & Thomson (1990; study of female prostitutes); Richwald et al. (1988; study of bathhouse users). In the Richwald study, men leaving bathhouses (in one-half of the cases, between the hours of midnight and 4 a.m.) were stopped and asked to fill out a questionnaire taking 15–30 minutes and asking detailed questions about sexual behavior and other personal matters. The intrusiveness was compounded unnecessarily by asking participants to sign consent forms, which then became the major threat to their anonymity and confidentiality.

public is concerned sufficiently about AIDS that many people are willing to suffer some embarrassment in answering personal questions (Taylor, 1993b), the fact remains that they *are* personal.

So too are questions about feelings and relationships. Illustrative of just how personal they are is an unpublished study conducted by Mark Small (Small, 1988) in which participants in a door-to-door survey identified personality testing as almost as invasive as nonconsensual videotaping of shoppers in store dressing rooms.

The problem of intrusiveness does not end with the data collection. Research about AIDS—even if it does not involve people who have HIV infection or whose behavior places them at high risk—may arouse sufficient anxiety and depression that the duty to minimize harm (APA, 1992, Std. 1.14 & Prin. E) requires that researchers do careful debriefing (cf. Std. 6.18) and that they take any other steps (e.g., provision of counseling or brief psychotherapy) that are necessary to remediate any harm that occurs.[9] Indeed, a focus on the circumstances that led a participant into research may itself be painful (see, e.g., Jenny et al., 1990, studying HIV seroprevalence among rape victims).

A study of the risk of sexually transmitted diseases, including HIV infection, among African American, adolescent (aged 13–19) users of crack cocaine illustrates the problems of intrusiveness in AIDS research (Fullilove, Fullilove, Bowser & Gross, 1990). Fullilove and colleagues presented an unusually detailed account of their recruitment and interview procedures, so it offers an excellent case for consideration of ethical issues in psychosocial research on AIDS:

> Network recruitment techniques were used to approach this elusive population. Interviewers [who were African American employees of local community service agencies "familiar with the local drug users and drug dealers"] recruited subjects from community centers located in neighborhoods known for crack use and crack sales and from the street corners where sales and use of crack occur openly. In such areas, passersby are

---

9. There may be other harms for which relatively detailed debriefing is required and which, therefore, entail a measure of intrusiveness beyond the research protocol itself. For example, studies that provide opportunities for homophobic, racist, or other prejudiced responses may require educational debriefing so that such attitudes are not inadvertently affirmed. Similar provisions may be necessary when interviews or questionnaires ask about adherence to inaccurate beliefs about AIDS. For an example of research on debriefing in an analogous context, see the study by Check and Malamuth (1984) on the effects of pornography research.

frequently stopped by crack dealers and asked if they are interested in buying "rock" (a slang term for crack) or, conversely, are asked by crack users who are interested in purchasing the drug where it can be bought. In either case, if interviewers were approached in this fashion (and when they deemed it to be safe), they identified themselves as workers who were conducting a survey about crack use. Initially, they asked those who approached them if they used crack. Those who admitted that they were users were then asked their age and if they would consent to participate in an anonymous survey about drug use and about sexual behavior.

If the invitation to participate was accepted, subjects were informed that they would not be identified by name, that their responses would be kept in strictest confidence, that they had the right to refuse to respond to any question that made them too uncomfortable (or that they found too personal), that they could terminate the interview at any time, and that they would be paid $10 for their participation. If agreement to participate was secured, the interview was conducted in any one of a variety of different private settings, ranging from the interviewer's car to an office at one of the community centers whose assistance we solicited in conducting the study. Those who refused or who indicated that they did not use crack were not interviewed but were asked to assist the interviewer in identifying potential subjects who were users.

Those who completed the interview were also asked to assist in identifying others who might participate in the study. Referrals were also made by community residents who were knowledgeable about the crack trade, by community workers from local churches or community-based organizations, and by counselors in local detention centers who worked with adolescent crack users and dealers. Interviewers reported that recruitment efforts resulted in 11 refusals, a 95% participation rate, with refusals being attributed almost exclusively to lack of time to commit to an interview.

To ensure that study subjects were in fact crack users (and not simply claiming to be crack users to obtain the $10 participation fee) interviewers used a number of verification techniques. These included the interviewer's direct observation of the respondent either using crack or selling crack, a referral from trusted community members who had direct knowledge of the respondent's crack use, or a referral by juvenile authorities (e.g., probation officers, community drug outreach workers, policemen, etc.) of adolescents with a history of crack-related offenses. (p. 852)

Without attempting to resolve the questions raised by this study, let us simply raise some of them:

— Through their direct observation of crack use or dealing and their presumable failure to interrupt such behavior or disclose it to authorities, the researchers, some might argue, became accomplices to violations of the law, however passively.[10] Did the researchers have a duty to act either to stop the illegal behavior or to "blow the whistle" on it?

— In some instances, the researchers learned about crack use through the interviews rather than, or in addition to, direct observation. Are researchers' duties different when illegal behavior is learned through a "confession" as opposed to witnessing it directly?

— If a grand jury or a district attorney subpoenaed a participant's data pertaining, for example, to an allegation of a violation of probation, should the researcher comply? Should the researcher seek in advance to protect the data against such a subpoena?

— Should the fact that most of the participants were minors affect the answers to the previous questions? What duty do researchers have to change self-injurious behavior of minors participating in their research? Should such an effort be undertaken even if participants do not request it? if they affirmatively object? How should concern about adolescent participants' welfare be balanced against concern for their privacy?

— Do the researchers owe any duty to the participants' parents, who apparently did not give permission for the research?[11] If you believe that the participants' interests would be protected better or at least as well by the preservation of confidentiality with respect to their parents, does it matter that parent-child relations may be addressed during the interviews? In studies of minors, especially those who have given independent consent to researchers, should researchers take care to minimize the intrusion on their parents' privacy? Should any other limits

10. For another study raising similar issues, see the ethnographic study of needle sharing in Rotterdam by Grund, Kaplan, and Adriaans (1991). Grund et al. engaged in "intense participant observation of addicts' self-administration of heroin and cocaine at dealing places, their homes, and public places" (p. 1603). They made detailed fieldnotes of 95 "rituals" (i.e., incidents of drug taking). These issues are raised not by way of suggesting that any researchers should have been charged with criminal conduct, but rather to underscore the fact that research relating to criminal conduct often raises potential legal (and corresponding ethical) problems. In fact, as we note in Chapter 5 just prior to the concluding section, a researcher's conduct in this context likely would not rise to a level where criminal liability would attach.

11. Of course, the omission of parental consent is itself questionable (see Grisso, 1992, and the relevant discussion in Chap. 2 of this volume).

be put on the content of interviews when parents have not given permission for their children's participation?

— Are there questions that are appropriate to pose to adult crack users, but that are too personal or upsetting to ask adolescent crack users?

— Was the snowball recruitment procedure (users who identify other potential participants) defensible? Should researchers who use such procedures require that the original participants obtain potential participants' permission to be contacted? Were the other recruitment procedures (e.g., direct approach to individuals when they were observed to use crack or when they were reported by friends or authorities to be users) unduly intrusive?

— What sort of debriefing should the researchers have undertaken? How deeply should the researchers have probed about the participants' reactions to the study? If the researchers believed that a particular participant had been disturbed by the interview, should they have contacted the youth's parents or other authorities?

— If the researchers learned that a thirteen-year-old was engaging in high-risk behavior and was essentially unsupervised or even encouraged by his or her parents to engage in such behavior, would the researchers have a duty to inform child protection authorities?

— If HIV-antibody testing had been part of the protocol, would the answers to any of the previous questions change?

In noting these questions, we do not intend to suggest that the study by Fullilove et al. is "unethical" and thus remarkable. Rather, the unusually clear description by Fullilove et al. of their methods enables us to raise questions that are rather widespread in AIDS research. These questions are not easy as a matter of ethics, and they are typically unclear as a matter of law.[12] An important point that they suggest is that ethical problems snowball: the decision that it is appropriate to contact youthful crack users to seek their involvement in research does not answer any of the other questions. That a particular procedure or scope of inquiry is not unduly intrusive is not implied by the conclusion that *some* research is justifiable.

The snowball occurs in reverse, too. Although the overall recruitment and design may be defensible, a particular problem (e.g., the scope of debriefing that is practical) may be so difficult that it cannot be resolved satisfactorily. In such an instance, the choice becomes one of avoidance of the

12. Some of the law relevant to the questions in the text is discussed in succeeding chapters.

ethical problem and, therefore, failure to undertake the research or acceptance of the problematic solution and a decision to conduct ethically and sometimes legally questionable research. In this instance, for example, is determination of the specific risk to adolescent crack users on the street—when, after all, it is already known that they *are* at risk—likely to produce sufficient new knowledge to warrant de facto complicity in the would-be participants' drug use?

As we have already stated, we raise this study as an exemplar of the complexity of ethical issues that arise in the context of research about AIDS. The issues involved in the study are unique neither to psychosocial research nor to AIDS research more broadly. Although some of the issues that arose in the context of the Fullilove et al. (1990) study were population-, question-, or approach-specific, most AIDS research is fraught with ethical concerns. Thus, in important ways, the study is quite typical.

The one answer to the questions that we have presented that is clear is that researchers have a duty to minimize the intrusiveness of their work. They should search for the most discreet means of recruitment, and they should ask the least probing questions that will elicit sufficient information to make the study worthwhile. In keeping with general advice that we will provide at the end of this chapter, researchers should also consult with other experts on the population of interest and with youth and other community members themselves to obtain diverse points of view about not only the ethical issues per se but also the means of resolving them, such as alternative means of participant recruitment.

Inflicted Information

A general strategy for decreasing intrusiveness is increasing choice. Consent does not abrogate the duty to minimize intrusiveness, but privacy is protected to the extent that participants feel fully in control of others' exploration into their personal affairs.

Although, as discussed in Chapter 2, federal research policy generally emphasizes informed consent, policymakers in the Public Health Service have been unwilling to carry this principle to its logical conclusion in research in which HIV antibody testing is part of the protocol. Federal policy (Office for Protection from Research Risks, 1984; Windom, 1988) provides that in all research that includes HIV testing and in which identifying information is kept, participants "must be informed of their own test results and provided with the opportunity to receive appropriate counseling. . . . Individuals may not be given the option 'not to know' the result, either at the time of consenting to be tested or thereafter" (Windom, 1988, p. 1).

The policy does provide limited exceptions. First, test results need not be disclosed to particular individuals when there are "compelling and immediate reasons" to justify the nondisclosure. An example of such a circumstance would be suicide risk. Second, Institutional Review Boards (IRBs) can waive the requirement of disclosure of HIV test results if "extremely valuable knowledge might be gained from research involving subjects who would be expected to refuse to learn their HIV antibody results." Such waivers must be reevaluated periodically by the IRB to determine whether nondisclosure is still justified in light of "the risk-benefit ratio to individuals, their partners, and society" (Windom, 1988, p. 2). Third, the policy leaves open the possibility of culturally specific risk-benefit ratios, so that nondisclosure may be justified in some research conducted at foreign sites.

The list of exceptions to unwanted disclosure is striking for the absence of consideration of participant autonomy and privacy. Although the policy itself does not provide rationales justifying it, it appears to be premised on the view of some commentators that "persons who are screened and whose seropositivity is confirmed have a moral obligation to learn that information" (Bayer, Levine & Wolf, 1986, p. 1770). Thus, the protection of society is believed to override any individual's own preferences.

Bayer and colleagues' view (apparently like the federal policy) was based on a fundamental—and questionable—empirical assumption that knowledge of a positive HIV antibody test, even if the participant desires not to know the results, often in itself will result in safer behavior. Bayer et al. acknowledged that there are empirical counterarguments:

1. Just as health care workers' risk of exposure to HIV can be minimized by "universal precautions," an individual's action to protect others from possible HIV infection does not require knowledge of his or her serostatus.

2. Knowledge of one's seropositivity "may be so psychologically devastating that the individual will suffer greatly without any benefits to himself or herself or additional benefits to others."

Although Bayer et al. recognized the speculative nature of their own assumption and the validity of the counterarguments, they asserted that the counterarguments bore little weight in the face of other empirical hypotheses:

1. The proponents of a right not to know "underestimate the power of denial and the difficulty of sustaining behavioral change in the absence of specific information."
2. Assuming that *some* people with HIV infection will engage in safer behavior only if they know their serostatus, "there is no way to discern in advance who of the infected people will modify their behavior without notification and who will not, much less who will be consistent in those changes."

Empirical research on the effects of HIV antibody testing and the factors involved in effective prevention of HIV infection lend general support to both proponents and opponents of a right not to know. Research has shown substantial risk reduction among gay men and IV drug users, regardless of whether they have been tested for HIV antibodies (Becker & Joseph, 1988; Des Jarlais & Friedman, 1988; Stall, Coates & Hoff, 1988). Moreover, most studies have shown greater risk reduction among individuals who have undergone testing and counseling and who have been found to be seropositive (Coates et al., 1988), although such a difference may reflect greater frequency of risk behaviors among people who become infected and therefore more room for change (see, e.g., McCusker et al., 1988).

Research on the emotional consequences of testing is scant, but the preponderance of data supports the common-sense view that a positive HIV antibody test induces depression and anxiety and that some people have serious mental health crises with heightened suicide risk (Coates et al., 1988; see, e.g., Joseph, Montgomery & Kirscht, 1987, and Marzuk et al., 1988). Research on the depressive effects of positive HIV antibody test results on blood donors suggests that such effects may be particularly pronounced in people who do not specifically seek testing (Cleary et al., 1993). Compelled counseling also may disturb *adaptive* denial that permits some people with life-threatening illnesses to cope with the dreadful reality that they face (Koocher & O'Malley, 1981).

Research on the emotional and behavioral effects of testing may not be directly apposite to the problem posed by the PHS policy, because the policy affects people who, but for their participation in research, would not be tested (or at least would not be tested as soon). At least two studies have examined the effects of a choice to receive HIV antibody test results in the context of a research protocol.

Between 1985 and 1987, participants in a large-scale study of the natural history of HIV infection among gay and bisexual men in the vicinity of Pittsburgh were offered the choice of knowing their HIV serostatus (Lyter, Valdiserri, Kingsley, Amoroso & Rinaldo, 1987). Sixty-one percent accepted the invitation, and 54 percent actually attended a results disclosure meeting. That almost one-half of the participants failed to accept the invitation for confidential test disclosure and counseling suggests that a requirement of disclosure of test results may constrict study samples substantially.

Those who accepted the invitation did not differ from those who formally declined (9 percent) in age, race, education, HIV serostatus, recent sexual behavior, attitudes about AIDS and risk reduction practices, or knowledge about HIV testing, local HIV seroprevalence, or risk-reduction practices. Both those who accepted and those who refused to receive their test results were substantially more likely to believe erroneously that they were infected than to err in the belief that they were not infected.

Participants who failed to respond to multiple invitations (30%) were somewhat younger on average, more likely to be nonwhite, and less likely to have a college degree, although the magnitude of such differences was small. The nonresponse group did not differ in rate of seropositivity from those who accepted or formally declined the invitation to receive their HIV antibody test results. Among those who formally declined and who gave a reason for doing so,[13] more than one-third identified fear of their psychological reaction to a positive test (inability to cope) as their most important reason.

Similar findings were recorded in a study conducted between 1984 and 1986 in the Baltimore-Washington area (Fox, Odaka, Brookmeyer & Polk, 1987). Two-thirds of the participants—all gay men—elected to learn their HIV serostatus. Those who chose to learn their result did not differ from those who refused in their age, race, number of sex partners, AIDS-related symptoms, or serostatus, although the refusers were more likely to be college-educated.

Six months after the disclosure of test results, the mean number of sexual partners and, in particular, of sexual partners with whom the participants had engaged in anal intercourse had declined among participants who had opted not to learn their serostatus, those who learned that they were seronegative, and those who had positive test results. These changes were *least* common among participants who had learned that they were

13. Twenty percent gave no reason.

infected with HIV. Participants aware of their seronegative status were slightly more likely than refusers to reduce their risky sexual behavior.

In short, although awareness of test results can have some positive effects, it also can have negative effects, and a change in behavior commonly but not universally occurs, regardless of the decision to receive test results. A requirement to receive test results is almost certain to narrow the sample,[14] although the bias in the sample may be more in emotional than in behavioral traits or demographic characteristics.

Ultimately, though, the issue is one of values. The key assumptions on both sides are essentially a priori. The observation that a person with HIV infection does not need to know his or her own serostatus to avoid exposure of others is true on its face. There is no logical necessity of knowledge of positive serostatus for either abstinence from sexual intercourse and needle sharing or "safer" sex (e.g., use of condoms) and IV drug use (e.g., use of needles cleaned with bleach).[15] Similarly, the opponents of a right to know will have their point of rebuttal about behavior change confirmed if *anyone* adopts safer behavior as a result of knowledge of his or her seropositivity. Intuition is enough to validate this limited assumption. (Of course, this assumption is one-sided; it ignores the possibility that some will choose riskier behavior, either because of undue confidence resulting from a negative test or bravado resulting from a positive test and a corollary belief that one cannot be harmed further.)

Bayer et al. and the PHS apparently judged the significance of individual autonomy less weighty in the face of "the disastrous consequences of HIV infection and the imperative of the harm principle" (Bayer et al., 1986, p. 1770).[16] In essence, they held that when the threat involved is grave, public safety trumps personal autonomy.

Even if the general conclusion is valid, it is unclear why it should result

14. Indicative of this effect is a study at a San Francisco obstetrics-gynecology clinic (cited by Coates et al., 1988) that showed 10–12 percent of women would avoid prenatal care or venereal disease treatment if HIV antibody testing were a condition of receipt of such services.

15. We use the term "safer" sex to acknowledge that some risks remain when high risk behavior is engaged in, even if steps are taken to minimize that risk. For example, many have advocated the use of household bleach as a means of eradicating the HIV virus in IV injection equipment. However, recent reports have suggested that such practices may not be as effective as once believed (e.g., "Community Alert," 1993 [reporting findings "that use of bleach is an imperfect approach to eradicate or inactivate HIV from injection equipment"]).

16. Bayer et al. (1986) defined the *harm principle* as the justification for "limitations on an individual's liberty to pursue personal goals and choices when others will be harmed by those activities" (p. 1769).

in a requirement that research participants learn their HIV-antibody test results when identifiable data are available. Very few suggest mandatory testing, even of people in "risk groups." Society generally has decided that the benefits of testing and personal disclosure of results do not justify their imposition except in limited contexts, and even those contexts are controversial. Why should research participants be any different?

In effect, the PHS policy results in research participants being rewarded for their altruism with *fewer* rights than individuals who do not participate! Such a policy of forced disclosure is no less disrespectful of autonomy and privacy than would be a policy of withholding personally relevant information such as the results of medical tests.

Of course, individuals who do not want to learn their serostatus can avoid doing so simply by refusing to participate in studies in which HIV testing is conducted and blood samples are identified. The federal policy thus does not abrogate autonomy altogether. Indeed, the fact that serostatus will be revealed must be disclosed in order to obtain informed consent.

Nonetheless, when the nonparticipants would not otherwise be required to learn their serostatus, it is unclear why it is desirable to limit study samples (by increased refusals) and thus to reduce the ability to generalize research results in largely unknown ways. Accordingly, we believe that the PHS policy is neither consistent with the public interest in development of knowledge about AIDS nor sufficiently respectful of participants' autonomy. The threats to the public interest and participants' autonomy have become somewhat less acute as calls for mandatory testing have abated, but as long as the policy remains, the threats persist. Therefore, we favor its rescission.

We acknowledge, though, that the case is somewhat less clear to us than it was at the time that the PHS policy was promulgated.[17] The difference is the availability of treatments that retard the development of symptoms among people who have HIV infections (e.g., Hirschel et al., 1991; Pape, Verdier & Johnson, 1989; State-of-the-Art Conference, 1990; Volberding et al., 1990). Therefore, knowledge of seropositivity now has

---

17. As a member of both the Task Force on Psychology and AIDS and the Committee for Protection of Human Participants in Research, one of us (Melton) was involved in extensive discussions of the PHS policy when it was promulgated. Both of those bodies under the governance of the American Psychological Association registered their strong opposition to the policy, which was communicated in a joint letter by the executive directors of the APA Public Interest and Science Directorates.

a benefit for asymptomatic HIV-positive individuals. In that regard, the question of the right not to know is illustrative of the general principle, discussed in Chapter 6, that public health law and policy evolve in tandem with scientific knowledge. Nonetheless, when individuals knowingly forego that potential benefit, we can think of no reason why the fact of research participation should lead to compulsory access to it.

International Research

AIDS is now a pandemic of global proportions. The numbers are staggering: as of early 1992, HIV infection had occurred in approximately 12.9 million people, about one-fifth (2.6 million) of whom had developed AIDS. Of those with AIDS, more than 95 percent had died (Tarantola & Mann, 1993). Two million people are estimated to have been infected by HIV in Thailand, Burma, and India in the past two years. The infection rate in Kampala, the capital of Uganda, may be near one in three (Goodgame, 1990). By the end of the decade, the number of people with HIV infection may reach nine figures—the vast majority of whom will be counted among residents of developing countries (Tarantola & Mann, 1993).

The catastrophic scope of the AIDS epidemic in parts of Africa and Asia poses special challenges. Most obviously, the cost in health care, social services, and lost productivity is an extraordinary burden for countries that often lack an extensive human service system and in which most people already live in poverty. The situation is complicated by the difficulty that developing countries face in purchasing treatments currently available, the differences between the epidemiology of HIV infection in the West and that in the Third World, the lack of an indigenous scientific infrastructure, and postcolonial skepticism about the motives and diligence of the West in responding to the crisis—factors that all point to the need to develop specialized programs, including regulatory mechanisms, for AIDS research.

The accomplishment of such a goal inevitably entwines researchers in international politics. This phenomenon has been present since the first years of the AIDS epidemic. Although the early onslaught of cases of AIDS occurred largely in the United States, the political context for attempts to understand the disease was complicated by the remarkably high incidence of AIDS among Haitian immigrants. The initial classification of Haitians as a risk group—a status that persisted until 1985 (Centers for Disease Control, 1985b)—heightened discrimination against a group already beleaguered and subsequently caught in major disputes about immigration policy. It also increased tension with the Haitian government, which was concerned about the effects of such stigma on international tourism and trade (Panem, 1984). Similar conflicts have occurred with some African countries, which have seen a decline of their fledgling tourist industry and which were offended by early speculation that HIV originated in African primates (Fortin, 1991).

Researchers now face two central dilemmas in their work on AIDS in the Third World. Perhaps the most poignant are those that deal with justice in the allocation of the risks and benefits of research. On the one hand, because of their limited resources and minimal regulatory system for research and health care, there is a risk of exploitation of people in developing countries. This possibility is given particular meaning by the fact that some African countries appear to be especially attractive sites for vaccine research, because the attack rates (i.e., incidence or rate of increase in new cases) are so enormous that there is much less likelihood than in most American communities that experimental vaccines will be "wasted" on, and risks incurred by, individuals who would have remained seronegative in any event. Additionally, the higher attack rates allow researchers to acquire information much more quickly through use of Third World samples. Although this phenomenon at least raises the possibility that developing countries will obtain medical means of containing the epidemic substantially earlier than would have occurred otherwise, it also opens the door to imposition on Third World peoples of risks that people in Western countries are unwilling to accept. On the other hand, the vast number of people with HIV infection in some countries in Asia and Africa suggests the need for a much more intensive research campaign than has occurred there yet.

The second major dilemma concerns the applicability of American professional norms and federal regulations to research conducted in the Third World. For example, is the application of conventional American procedures for informed consent a form of ethnocentric "ethical imperialism" that is borne of arrogant disregard of indigenous norms, or is such an approach indicative of a partnership with local hosts that is based on mutual respect—a desire to avoid cutting corners when people's dignity is at stake?

The general answer to the dilemma depends in part on factual anthropological assumptions. Some commentators (e.g., Barry, 1988) claim that personhood (at least as the concept is understood in the West) is alien to many sub-Saharan cultures and that insistence on informed consent may seem not only nonsensical but also offensive to African participants whose worldview focuses more on community (tribe) than on individuality. Others (e.g., Angell, 1988) note that the fundamental tenets in research ethics are not "American" in that they are present in a number of international agreements (see Melton, 1992), which commonly are even more restrictive than U.S. federal research regulations and which typically are recognized throughout the world. Such commentators argue further that the establishment of less stringent standards for research regulation in the name of cultural sensitivity ironically may lead to exploitation of Third World populations.

Commenting on this dilemma, Goodgame (1990) noted that the cultural expectation in Uganda, where he conducts clinical research, is that the doctor will not discuss patients' diagnoses and treatments with them. At the same time, the official policy of the Ugandan government, which is attempting to increase individual responsibility, is that people with HIV infections should be informed so that they can take appropriate precautions. Goodgame (1990, p. 387) concluded that clinical experience shows that "there are many more similarities than differences" in the psychological response of Ugandan and American patients. For most patients, regardless of culture, the diagnosis of HIV infection or AIDS is distressing, but frank and caring discussion of the situation offers some reassurance.

The dilemmas of AIDS research in the Third World are given meaning when one considers the magnitude of the discrepancies between everyday life for many research participants in that context and for those even in some of the most endangered Western communities. For example, Kreiss et al. (1986) studied seroprevalence and behavior epidemiology among prostitutes in Nairobi, Kenya, one sample of whom reported nearly 1,000 sexual encounters per year for about 50 cents each. Bertrand et al. (1991) examined sexual behavior, condom use, and knowledge about AIDS among 3,000 people in Zaire, each of whom was interviewed in detail about intimate behavior. Only about one-tenth of the sample lived in homes with indoor plumbing, and only about one-half owned a radio. Many of the respondents reported not only a lack of condom use but also a belief that effective vaccines and treatments are available for AIDS.

In the end, the answer to the controversy may be one of simple respect and common sense. As Barry (1988) noted, "when language barriers exist and such concepts as germ theory or viral agents are alien, a description of an AIDS-related investigation, even a simple seroprevalence study, becomes difficult to relay to participants" (p. 1084). The issue is not one of conformity to rituals of informed consent (almost no one seriously argues that the answer to ethical problems in research in the Third World is the provision of forms to people unaccustomed to them and often poorly educated), but instead adherence to the spirit that underlies that doctrine as well as notions of distributive justice. Concern for dignity is a human universal, but sensible and sensitive researchers will enlist local leaders in finding ways to communicate that concern.

That conclusion, which admittedly may sound easier than it is, does not obviate the fact that protection of Third World people from undue risk or simple commercial exploitation may be necessary as the clamor builds for human trials of vaccines for AIDS. Although the establishment of local watchdog and advisory groups may help, the situation is complicated because some of the countries in which trials are likely to occur earliest have authoritarian governments that may have agendas other than the promotion of social welfare and protection of individual dignity. The need is clear for Western and indigenous teams that would combine expertise in scientific, cultural, ethical, and political matters.

Duties to and for Research Assistants

Discussions of research ethics typically center on the welfare of participants, as balanced against various societal concerns. As we pointed out at the beginning of this chapter, such debates often miss the mark by ignoring the self-interest of the researcher. Another often missing aspect of the researcher's side of the balancing test is the role played by individuals on the research team other than the principal investigator (PI).

This underemphasized role has received some attention in the context of investigations of scientific fraud. When PIs delegate data observation, recording, and analysis, questions may arise about their culpability for misrepresentations made by their assistants without their knowledge. In that regard, the Ethical Principles of Psychologists (American Psychological Association, 1992) place responsibility squarely with the PI: "Psychologists are responsible for the ethical conduct of research conducted by them or by others under their supervision or control" (Std. 6.07[b]).

More specifically germane to AIDS research and directly relevant to this chapter, researchers bear responsibility for ensuring that their assistants are sufficiently well trained to show appropriate sensitivity to the norms of the groups they are studying.[18] This obligation of sensitivity, of

---

18. The Ethical Principles provide that "assistants are permitted to perform only those tasks for which they are appropriately trained and prepared" (American Psychological Association, 1992, Std. 6.07 [c]). Although this standard was probably based on a desire to

course, applies with equal force to biomedical and other types of research. Assistants must also show proper respect for participant privacy, and researchers must design research procedures and staff training that minimize the potential for leaks of confidential information.

Another aspect of the researcher-assistant relationship that may arise in AIDS research relates to assistants' safety. Although the risk to staff involved in AIDS clinical research is extremely low, it is not zero when venipuncture is part of the protocol (see Anonymous, 1990, reporting a house officer's seroconversion, and National Institute for Occupational Safety and Health, 1989, describing precautions recommended for health care workers). It has been estimated that approximately 0.3–0.4 percent of cases of accidental exposure to HIV as a result of needle-stick injuries result in seroconversion (Becker, Cone & Gerberding, 1989; Henderson et al., 1990).[19]

A recent federal decision suggests that researchers have a duty to warn their assistants about dangers that they may encounter and presumably to offer means (e.g., training about CDC guidelines; provision of rubber gloves) of abating them. In *Andrulonis v. United States* I (1991), a state bacteriologist supervised by a federal scientist contracted rabies as a result of leaky laboratory equipment. Although the Circuit Court of Appeals noted that the imposition of a duty to warn research staff about potential hazards incurred in their work "may tend to chill the collegial atmosphere of the scientific community" (p. 1221), it concluded that staff "should not have to bear the financial burdens in addition to the personal risks that accompany the quest for scientific advancement" (p. 1221). Accordingly, it awarded damages to the injured bacteriologist.

Andrulonis should not be read so broadly that it stands for a judicial mandate for hysteria. As discussed in the remainder of this chapter, a basic contribution of science to AIDS policy should be the abatement of undue fear. Nonetheless, researchers who study HIV-infected blood samples should be advised that, to minimize the risk of harm and their own or their institution's liability, they should do more than just assume that assistants

---

avoid risk of harm to participants and society, it could also reasonably be read to imply a responsibility to avoid danger to assistants who might undertake tasks that carry personal risk but for which they have not been trained.

19. These figures may actually overrepresent the risk posed to research assistants, as contrasted with clinical service providers. This is because, in research settings, circumstances are likely to be more controlled, and there is a higher likelihood that "universal" or other precautions will be undertaken.

are taking common-sense precautions that were included in their training. Staff should be provided with frequent and explicit reminders about risks (even if small) that they face and means of avoiding such risks.

The Competence of Researchers

> Psychologists conduct research competently and with due concern for the dignity and welfare of the participants. (APA, 1992, Std. 6.07[a])[20]

Conceptually, the mixture in a single standard of the duties of competence (fidelity to role), respect for persons, and beneficence is an odd combination. Although those duties need not conflict, they involve diverse obligations that, for coherence, might have been separated and matched with more clearly similar responsibilities.

In the context of AIDS research, however, competence, respect, and beneficence fit neatly, because the major pitfalls in such work emanate from a lack of sensitivity to cultural differences and the situation in which people with HIV infection and those at risk for it find themselves. In a section of the Ethical Principles that is derived from discussion of the issues in AIDS research, psychologists are obliged to "consult those with expertise concerning any special population under investigation or most likely to be affected" (APA, 1992, Std. 6.07[d]; see also Prin. D and Std. 1.08).

In that regard, the record of health care professionals in handling the stigma attached to people with AIDS and to groups that have high rates of HIV infection has been less than stellar. Clinicians have indicated much less willingness to interact with people with AIDS than with people with leukemia (Kelly, St. Lawrence, Hood, Smith & Cook, 1987b). Large proportions of physicians would decline treating HIV-infected patients if they could, many admit to homophobic attitudes, and most say that they lack information needed to treat patients with AIDS (Adler, 1992b). Unfortunately, some evidence suggests that the next generation of physicians will also harbor negative attitudes toward AIDS (Kelly, St. Lawrence, Hood, Smith & Cook, 1987a).

Researchers cannot blithely attribute such prejudices to those whose affinity is more for practice than for science. As one commentator noted, the AIDS epidemic has been remarkable for "the appearance in prestigious

---

20. An obligation to stay within one's competence in research is also found in Principle A and Standards 1.04 and 6.06(a). Standard 6.06(a) requires specifically that researchers adhere to "recognized standards of scientific competence and ethical research," a point that is reiterated in Standard 6.08.

medical journals of complaints, whines, and pleas for understanding from doctors worried about contamination and ruination" (Bosk & Frader, 1991, p. 160, citations omitted[21]). Moreover, as discussed in Chapter 6, the "other epidemic"—the epidemic of fear—has peaked after thoughtless public announcements of journal articles (sometimes with accompanying supportive editorials) and books that contained mistaken conclusions by prestigious scientists.

Most directly to the point, research (e.g., Bennett et al., 1989; Lewis, Freeman & Corey, 1987) indicates that skill in AIDS-related practice is correlated with health care professionals' comfort and experience in working with people in behavior risk groups (see Robiner, Parker, Ohnsorg & Strike, 1993, for a review). Although we are unaware of comparable research on the competence of AIDS researchers, the need to frame questions and draw conclusions in the context of various cultures and groups suggests that the relationship between competence in AIDS-related research and sensitivity to the norms and experience of affected groups may be even stronger.[22]

The message is clear. Not only formal study but also consultation with affected groups—a point about which more will be said—is critical to research that is both scientifically valid and ethically sound. Fortunately, research suggests that affirmative efforts to learn more about AIDS and the groups that it has affected most profoundly do result in both increased

21. The citations were from the journals of the American, British, and Canadian medical associations.

22. As a practical matter, without a relationship of trust between researchers and the affected community, the ability to generalize research results is likely to be compromised by (a) high rates of refusals and attrition in the sample and (b) less than full honesty in response to sensitive but key questions. In this regard, it is noteworthy that the dropout rate in clinical research on AIDS has been unusually high, which has led some medical research groups to add psychologists to their team to assist in working with participants (Adler, 1992c). See Merigan (1989) for a personal account of the issues that have been encountered by the AIDS Clinical Trials Group. Health care professionals themselves sometimes have used their knowledge of side effects to determine the likely group membership of their patients involved in purportedly double-blind clinical trials (see White, Kando, Park, Waternaux & Brown, 1992), and at other times they have lied about patients' health status to ensure their participation in such trials (Novick, 1990b). Such subversion of research designs, whether by participants or their physicians, in the long run serves neither the participants themselves nor society. For example, it results in unduly conservative research findings and, accordingly, prolongs clinical trials unnecessarily.

For a review of the issues that arose in the initial clinical trial of zidovudine (AZT; then known as azidothymidine; Fischl et al., 1987) and its early trial termination and subsequent approval by the Food and Drug Administration, see Brook (1987), Marwick (1987), Melton, Levine, Koocher, Rosenthal & Thompson (1988), and Windom (1986).

knowledge and greater comfort in dealing with the topic (Robiner et al., 1993).

Decision Making amid Uncertainty

Coping with Ambiguity

AIDS-related ethical problems are too complex to permit cookbook solutions (like removal of identifying information in research). Not only do such problems demand *thinking* ethically (as well as behaving in consonance with the strictures of ethical codes), but they also commonly will result at best in "balanced" decisions that do not fully accommodate all of the legitimate and even compelling interests. Just as there may be no *easy* solutions to ethical problems related to AIDS, there sometimes may be no *satisfactory* solutions. (Melton, 1991a, p. 563, emphasis added)

The complexity is exacerbated by the fact that ethical problems in AIDS research often are a product in part of uncertainty about the natural history of HIV infection and the technology of AIDS prevention and treatment. Therefore, the ethical calculus is changing constantly—uncertainty that is likely to become even more salient as the difficult dilemmas surrounding human trials of AIDS vaccines approach ("Federal Researcher Predicts," 1992; Marks, 1992; Osmond, 1992; Taylor, 1993a).

Amid empirical uncertainty and complex and often conflicting interests, the ethical and legal problems involved in AIDS research are both difficult and profound, and few researchers have had formal tutelage in their analysis. Fewer still were instructed in graduate, medical, or public health school about how to resolve the political conflicts that emerge from the ethical quagmire in which AIDS researchers often find themselves. Although the scientific enterprise is pushed ahead by creativity, its method is one of painstaking investigation, and its interpretive style is conservative and precise. (In contrast, one can be sure that politicians and community leaders rarely wait to see whether a magical p value is achieved before they draw conclusions about either social reality or a plan of action.)

The instinct of researchers who encounter the dilemmas involved in AIDS research is thus likely to be to act in a cautious, step-by-step manner. Such an ethically, politically, and scientifically complex area seems to demand an approach even more deliberate and contemplative than is the norm.

Regardless, the stakes are sufficiently high and the emotion resulting from them sufficiently intense that the desire for sober reflection may seem to be no more than wishful thinking. When delay means that more people may die, thoughtfulness is a luxury. At the same time, however, thoughtlessness heightens the risk of mistakes that may cause serious harm to many people. Carelessness may also result in insensitivity (even if inadvertent) that not only may be offensive to some groups or individuals but also may increase distrust of the research establishment to a point that the development of critically important knowledge is impeded.

Peer Consultation

To promote thoughtful inquiry in ethically problematic areas of study, both the Ethical Principles of Psychologists (APA, 1992, Std. 6.06[c]) and the federal regulations on research require consultation at least with peers and, to some extent, affected groups (cf. APA, 1992, Std. 6.08, requiring cooperation with federal regulatory bodies in the conduct of research). The entity established by federal regulations that is charged with peer review is the Institutional Review Board (IRB), now a fixture in all universities and agencies receiving federal funds for research.

IRB review of research projects is structured to facilitate the consideration of central ethical duties (e.g., Protection of Human Subjects, 45 C.F.R. § 46.111[a]), 1992 [Health and Human Services]):

— risks to participants must be minimized;
— risks to participants that are present must be reasonable in relation to anticipated benefits;
— the selection of participants must be equitable;
— information about material facts must be disclosed, and voluntary consent must be provided;
— provisions must be made for continuing risk-benefit analysis after some data are collected, to ensure that the design is consistent with participants' welfare;
— provisions must be made to protect the privacy of participants and to maintain the confidentiality of data;
— additional safeguards of participants' interests must be provided when, as in much AIDS research, they are especially vulnerable to coercion or undue influence (45 C.F.R. § 46.111[b]).

The effectiveness of IRBs as teams for consultation may be hampered, however, by this legalistic approach. Because IRBs are charged with deciding whether research can be conducted, they often seem to engage in checking off boxes (e.g., is a particular element included in a consent form?) instead of assisting in resolving critical ethical problems.

If the consultation function is to be fulfilled, the composition of the IRB becomes critical, so that the diverse interests involved in research on AIDS and other sensitive topics are represented. The federal rules require that the IRB contain representatives of diverse professions and ethnic backgrounds. In addition, if an IRB regularly reviews research that involves a vulnerable category of participants (e.g., IV drug users), the IRB must include at least one member who is primarily concerned with advocacy for those participants (45 C.F.R. § 46.107[a]). The IRB also may invite individuals with competence in special areas to assist in the review of complex issues (as often occur in AIDS research) (45 C.F.R. § 46.107[f]).

In short, IRBs may potentially serve the function of peer (or community) consultant, but the process of IRB review and the membership of the IRB do not necessarily lend themselves to thoughtful exploration by the IRB of the issues in collaboration with the researchers. Researchers may need to make a deliberate effort to seek the advice of other professionals in the area as well as the community of potential participants.

Community Consultation

Standard 6.07(d) of the Ethical Principles (APA, 1992) requires the consultation of experts about special populations involved in research; it does not specify that they be representatives of such populations. Although not excluding consultation with "experts," direct consultation with the communities that are likely to be affected by research is probably the optimal means of sensitization to ethical problems in research and to the development of ways of resolving them.

It cannot be assumed that participants would assess risks and benefits in the same ways that researchers and IRBs do. For example, almost all staff but only 50 percent of patients in methadone maintenance clinics in Harlem believed that clinic nurses and counselors should be informed about patients' HIV status (Curtis et al., 1989). Interestingly, Curtis et al. asked patients but not staff whether they knew their own HIV status, because such a question was "too intrusive" on the privacy of staff—but presumably not of patients! Similarly, questionnaires were administered anonymously to staff, but patients were asked to sign their names.

Building from concerns about such incidents, the establishment of a community forum for consultation with participant populations (e.g., gay men) or their surrogates (e.g., advocates for affected groups when they are unable to speak for themselves; people of a background similar to those who will be asked to participate in the research) has become a widely accepted approach to AIDS research (see, e.g., Levine, Dubler & Levine, 1991; Melton et al., 1988; Valdiserri, Tama & Ho, 1988). The Centers for Disease Control recently embraced the community consultation model with regard to AIDS prevention efforts. New rules that went into force on January 1, 1994 regulate the distribution of funds. They require grantees to establish community planning groups to develop prevention plans and assess local needs. "These planning groups must include representatives of the HIV-affected population and HIV organizations as well as state and local health officials . . ." (Freiburg, 1994, p. 32). Such an approach signals an honest attempt by researchers to form a partnership with participants and to take their concerns seriously in an effort to ensure justice. In that sense, the process itself may be as important as the substance of the decisions that are made in ensuring that the use of participants will not be unfair or cavalier.

Community consultation is not a panacea. After all, participants themselves often have conflicting interests, and loud voices may suppress some points of view. However, such problems are typically not intractable (see Melton et al., 1988, for practical suggestions derived from psychological research and theory relevant to community consultation). Most important, if taken seriously, community consultation is a check on researchers' self-interest and a means of dramatically and collegially identifying the interests at stake in AIDS research.

Chapter 2

INFORMED CONSENT

The principle of autonomy states that each person is in charge of his or her own body, life and vision. There is a strong relationship between this concept and personal "liberty" or privacy. The idea of autonomy is often alternatively expressed as respect for persons.

A. Novick, "May a Human Subject Waive the Right to be Treated as a Human Subject?"

At its core, the principle underlying informed consent is relatively simple: people should not be allowed to meddle in other people's lives unless the latter have agreed to such meddling after having been informed of what the meddling entails. Of course, there are questions at the periphery. These relate to issues such as the precise point at which conduct becomes meddlesome or who may or may not agree to it. Thus, informed consent is a process that expresses respect for the dignity and autonomy of other persons.

The ethical principle of respect for persons is the most fundamental requirement for informed consent (e.g., American Psychological Association [APA], 1992, Preamble and Principle [Prin.] D). The provision of relevant information and solicitation of knowing, competent, voluntary consent to AIDS research recognizes the autonomy of potential participants and attempts to "humanize" the relationship between researcher and participant (Katz, 1984), in addition to satisfying legal requirements. Such a theory also has found expression in federal regulations for informed consent in research and has sparked abundant commentary (e.g., Protection of Human Subjects, 45 C.F.R. part 46, 1992; Annas, Glantz & Katz, 1977; Barber, Lally, Makaruska & Sullivan, 1973; Gray, 1975; Katz, 1972; see Bower & de Gasparis, 1978, for an annotated bibliography relating to informed consent and other ethical issues in social research).

Recently, this discourse has produced many publications on the hotly debated topic of AIDS, resulting in guidelines and commentary on informed consent in AIDS research. Informed consent in AIDS research is particularly important for several reasons. First, despite all of the legal means by which privacy is protected (see Chap. 5,), none provides the majority of AIDS researchers with absolute protection against compelled or "voluntary" disclosures of confidential information. Second, the severity of potential harm arising from the disclosure of AIDS research-related information is considerable (see Chap. 3). Thus, when ostensibly confidential information is to be collected and retained by AIDS researchers, it is important that participants and/or their parents or guardians be fully informed of the associated disclosure risks, including when such information may be disclosed without consent and to whom the disclosures may be made (e.g., APA, 1992, Prin. 5.01). Third, as is often the case with research, direct benefits generally do not accrue to participants in AIDS research. Thus, researchers cannot rely on the beneficial quality of the research to override ethical considerations. Fourth, pediatric AIDS research is increasing, thus intensifying the need for informed consent procedures that are tailored to counteract the vulnerabilities of minor-aged participants. Finally, the seriousness of AIDS and the absence of a cure lead to variable states of desperation among people with AIDS. To guard against exploitation, investigators must apprise them fully of the distinction between medical procedures related to treatment and those related to research. Such appraisal should occur within the context of acquiring informed consent.

Because the acquisition of informed consent is both an essential prerequisite for ethical research and typically the first opportunity for researchers to behave in ways that will affect participants, it is not surprising that the issue occupies a central role in discussions of ethics in research. Ideally, research should proceed only after informed consent has been obtained whenever that research potentially places participants in a position in which they otherwise would not have been. Typically, the key considerations should be the wishes of the prospective participants and not any inherent value that might be ascribed to the research. In important ways, the relative merits of the research are irrelevant.

To be sure, research has benefited humankind tremendously. However, the principle of informed consent ensures that those benefits are not obtained at the expense of an unwilling few. As the Ninth Circuit Court of Appeals noted some years ago in the different context of labor union grievances, "The needs of the many do not always outweigh the needs of the few, or the one" (*Banks v. Bethlehem Steel Corp.*, 1989, p. 1443). No matter how beneficial knowledge would be regarding the effects of hypothermia or the etiology of syphilis, few would argue that those benefits would justify the experimentation by Nazis several decades ago in Germany or the actions of researchers more recently in Tuskegee (e.g., Thomas & Quinn, 1991).

That prospective participants themselves may benefit from research participation does not obviate the need for informed consent. Because they often are at once in desperate need of treatment and at a heightened risk of having impairments which may impede rational decision making, people with mental illnesses who are involuntarily committed comprise perhaps the clearest class of people for whom informed consent might arguably be dispensed with. Despite this, courts have held consistently that even individuals who have been committed retain sufficient residual autonomy to decide for themselves whether to submit to treatment. In *Washington v. Harper* (1990, pp. 221–222), for example, the United States Supreme Court observed that the inmate petitioner "possesse[d] a significant liberty interest in avoiding the unwanted administration of antipsychotic drugs under the Due Process Clause of the Fourteenth Amendment." Because mentally ill and dangerous prison inmates retain their constitutional right to make decisions regarding treatment, it would be difficult for researchers to argue that prospective research participants in other contexts do not retain similar control over their lives.

The need for acquisition of informed consent is perhaps best exemplified by the development of the Nuremburg Code, which was promulgated in response to Nazi physicians' outrageous experiments on concentration camp prisoners (e.g., *United States v. Brandt,* 1948). The Nuremburg Code prohibits any research that involves participants who have not given fully informed consent. Thus, it bars any research involving persons who, because of immaturity or mental disability, are incompetent to consent to research. It also bars any research using deception or incomplete disclosure. The Nuremburg Code remains the most comprehensive, and perhaps the most restrictive, statement of law relative to informed consent in the conduct of research.

In its exclusion of *any* nonconsensual research, the Nuremburg Code is unduly restrictive, even though such a prohibition was understandable in the context within which it was generated. Two issues arise. First, people with debilitating illnesses, such as AIDS (especially when patients are demented or hospitalized), would never profit from research if independent, competent consent was always required. Neither would young children. Second, although the doctrine of informed consent is primarily intended to protect autonomy, rigorous assurance of competence and voluntariness works in the opposite direction by denying "vulnerable" populations—including people with AIDS—the right to make important personal choices. As discussed in Chapter 1, such "protection" is particularly questionable when its effect is to deny access to experimental treatments when no effective, FDA-approved treatment is available (see Nichols, 1991). Moreover, the assumptions of incompetence and involuntariness themselves may reflect biases that are not consistent with empirical findings (see, e.g., Grisso, in press; Melton & Stanley, in press).

In addition to the Nuremburg Code, professional associations have emphasized the importance of informed consent by promulgating guidelines on informed consent for their disciplines.[1] Winslade and Ross (1985) provided a detailed discussion of the manner in which these and other professional codes strive to protect privacy.

Investigators and Institutional Review Boards (IRBs) have relied increasingly on informed consent procedures to resolve many of the ethical and legal dilemmas that are insufficiently resolved by other means (Katz, 1972, 1978; Meisel, 1977). The assumption is that informed assumption of risks or acquiescence to wrongs eliminates or at least mitigates the responsibility of investigators for questionable practices. Many commentators have questioned, however, whether reliance on informed consent procedures can produce the results that investigators intend (Fellner & Marshall, 1970; Gray, 1975; Lidz, 1977).

In this chapter we present and discuss the legal issues associated with the informed consent process. Although many researchers equate the acquisition of informed consent with the signing of a consent form, the receipt of signatures is only one consideration in the informed consent process. The consent form does not conclude the process; it only serves as evidence that adequate information has been provided to participants. Legally, a signature on an informed consent form creates only a prima facie case; that is, demonstrating that a participant signed the form merely shifts the burden of proving the case to the party alleging there was no consent. Thus, legal inquiry into whether consent actually was obtained does not end with evidence that a form was signed (e.g., Lidz & Roth, 1983).

The entire informed consent process involves, among other things, giving research participants adequate information concerning the study,

1. Exemplars include: the American Anthropological Association (1971), the American Medical Association (1966), the American Psychological Association (1992), the American Sociological Association (1971), the Declaration of Helsinki (1964), and the Society for Research in Child Development (1973).

providing adequate opportunity for participants to consider all options, responding to participants' questions, ensuring that they have comprehended the information and that they are competent to consent, and obtaining participants' voluntary consent to participation (e.g., Food and Drug Administration [FDA], 1989c).

The informed consent process cannot be understood or conducted adequately if limited to a legal inquiry of required informed consent components. The legal requirements for informed consent are not clear. Rather, they offer vague goals, leaving professional associations, IRBs, and individual researchers to clarify the method and route to compliance with the relevant regulations. Thus, the question of whether legal requirements for informed consent have been satisfied will be answered by common sense, formal ethical guidelines, professional recommendations, and relevant research findings concerning informed consent. Our discussion of the law of informed consent, of course, can offer no more guidance than does the law itself. Consequently, conspicuously absent will be specific guidelines in the form of "recipes" for informed consent forms. Such an approach would not only be inadequate, but would also minimize the complexity of the issues and interests at stake. Instead, the information that follows is offered to sensitize researchers to the issues involved and to provide a framework that researchers can apply to their own work.

Informed consent requirements for DHHS, the FDA, and common regulations (Protection of Human Subjects, 1992, 1993 [agencies listed]) are virtually the same. Therefore, we will discuss current DHHS regulations unless provisions differ in substantial ways. Legal regulations and ethical guidelines for the informed consent process may be viewed as consisting of four major components: (a) the disclosure of relevant information; (b) voluntariness; (c) the procedures for obtaining informed consent (e.g., comprehensibility and confidentiality); and (d) the identity of individuals with power of consent, permission, or assent (sections pertaining, e.g., to research involving state wards; research in foreign countries; and research involving participants of uncertain competence).

Required Disclosures

Description of Research

The basic requirement for informed consent is the presentation of whatever information may be relevant to a potential participant's decision whether to participate (e.g., APA, 1992, Standard [Std.] 6.11[b]; Protection of Human Subjects, 45 C.F.R. § 46.116, 1992 [Health and Human Services]). Thus, the researcher must outline why the study is being conducted and explain the potential benefit to society or participants, describe the research procedure, including any risks that may be involved, and supply any other information relevant to the decision of whether participation is worth the investment of time and assumption of risk. (This section applies primarily to adult participants, parents, or guardians. Special informed consent requirements for children are discussed below in the section entitled "Procedures for Obtaining Informed Consent.")

Specifically, the DHHS federal regulations require "a statement that the study involves research, an explanation of the purposes of the research and the expected duration of the subject's participation, a description of the procedures to be followed, and identification of any procedures that are experimental" (§ 46.116[a][1]).

Within this disclosure of information, the difference between treatment and research procedures must be made absolutely clear. In research that does not involve participants who are also clients or patients, this distinction is perhaps unnecessary, but the researcher should disclose the fact that research is being conducted, however apparently obvious that fact may be. In most medical research and the majority of AIDS research, the distinction between a treatment procedure and a research procedure is difficult for many patient-participants to discern. In particular, AIDS drug trial research is very likely to be perceived by potential participants with AIDS as holding some promise for improvement, despite the fact that the untested drug may not only be unhelpful, but harmful.

Lidz and Roth (1983) investigated patient-participants' understanding of a procedure's research status and the consent procedure used to inform them in a clinical research project. The research was a double-blind placebo study in which the investigators endeavored to use sleep electroencephalograph (EEG) studies to predict which patient-participants would respond positively to a particular drug. It involved the double-blind assignment of patient-participants to either placebo or drug-receiving categories and nightly monitoring of their sleep with EEG machines.

The major risks associated with the EEG study were related to the failure to receive any drug at all (placebo condition) or receipt of the drug in amounts that were not tailored to their particular needs. The authors reported that the staff did their best to explain the consent form carefully to the patient-participants. Following their signing of the consent form, they were given the final part of the two-part consent form. Finally, they were interviewed in depth by the psychiatrist on staff. The videotaped interview averaged about three-quarters of an hour and included all of the questions on the second part of the consent form as well as a series of other questions designed to uncover the patient's global understanding of the various issues associated with the decision. Only ten of the nineteen patient-participants were able to make a consistent distinction between research and treatment/diagnosis. The nine individuals who were unable to make the distinction conceptualized the research procedure as part of either treatment or diagnostic testing. Lidz and Roth reported that when these patient-participants were asked the purpose of the research, they responded with some variation of "It's to help make me better"—clearly indicating that they viewed the therapeutically neutral research as treatment.

The authors concluded that the key distinction between the two groups was an understanding of the concept of research. Patient-participants without any such appreciation did not consider the possibility that their doctors would do something that might not be in their best interest; they were found to show considerable creativity in construing nontherapeutic research procedures as therapeutic and in their interest after all.

With only one exception, the patient-participants seemed to have volunteered for the research project because they were convinced that it was somehow better to be on the research ward and in the research project than to be treated elsewhere. Uniformly, they believed that the doctor-investigators were there primarily to treat them. Although fully one-half of the subjects could describe the difference between treatment and research, they persisted in their belief that the research would make their treatment better. These patient-participants did not seem to understand that the research design sometimes forced the doctor-investigators to do something that may not have been in their best interests. They saw the research as an experimental treatment for them. Most of the patient-participants viewed the doctors' greater technical expertise as giving them the right to decide whether the patient should participate in the research. Thus, they tended to see the consent form as a formality that followed the decision, not as providing information on which to base a decision.

The patient-participants' apprehension difficulties could not be attributed simply to an inadequate informed consent form. A review of the videotaped interviews indicated that the misunderstandings were deep-seated and required a drastic revision of the entire informed consent process. The whole notion of the clinician-investigator had to be explained to the patients. Lidz and Roth reported that the patients almost had to be forced to understand that what the doctor was proposing was not necessarily the best or quickest treatment and that the compensations that were proposed did not do away with these limitations. The participants' belief that the doctor would look out for their best interest had to be challenged significantly for them to understand the decision fully.

Because of the lethal nature of AIDS, the dynamic described by Lidz and Roth may be especially problematic. People with HIV infection are often desperate for a cure or an effective means of ameliorating symptoms. This desperation may lead to an increased likelihood of confusion of research with treatment. This heightened vulnerability of people with AIDS thus creates a duty to be vigilant in ensuring that research participants understand the nature of their participation.

Description of Harmful Effects

Federal regulations require researchers to disclose to potential participants any reasonably foreseeable risks or discomforts directly or indirectly resulting from participation in the project (Protection of Human Subjects, 45 C.F.R. § 46.116[a][1], 1992 [Health and Human Services]). The knowledge of potential risks to AIDS research participants is an essential ingredient for reaching an informed decision concerning participation in the research. Although the specific risks potentially incurred by participating in research vary widely with each project (e.g., Gray, 1989; Gray & Melton, 1985), research on AIDS generally includes at least those risks resulting from breaches of confidentiality.

As the APA principles expressly require (1992, Std. 5.01), potential participants must be informed about the circumstances for which confidentiality might be limited. Researchers, in designing informed consent procedures, must attend carefully to the question of whether particular risks are sufficiently great to warrant discussion. For example, it is unlikely that anyone will have occasion to subpoena research data. Moreover, in the event that such data are subpoenaed, the individual from whom the data are subpoenaed probably will have sufficient opportunity to provide the data in a format that precludes identification of participants, at least with those studies involving a large number of subjects (see Chap. 3). Thus, researchers should be wary of providing lengthy descriptions of the negative consequences of events with remote probabilities.

The Lambda Legal Defense and Education Fund (1984, p. 27) stated that any possible risks associated with the potential disclosure of identifying information should be disclosed to AIDS research participants before participation. Such a disclosure should include, but is not limited to, any potential risks associated with (a) unauthorized releases of information to: insurance companies, employers, or the military; (b) criminal liability; (c) release to other possible government agencies (e.g., PHS, FDA); (d) HIV, abuse/neglect, and any other state or federal reporting requirements; and (e) subpoenas.

There are, of course, countervailing pressures that work against complete honesty. For instance, if all possible harmful effects were discussed in detail, it is possible that few people would be willing to participate. Ethically, this should be of concern only to the extent that participants are unduly alarmed or confused by a complex list of risks and benefits. If prospective participants were unduly alarmed, the principle of Social Responsibility would be violated doubly (APA, 1992, Prin. F). The good of the individual would be compromised by unnecessary stress, and social welfare would be adversely affected by the difficulty in recruiting participants and, therefore, in conducting research. Insofar as the concerns of participants are justified, the solution should be to diminish risk, not to hide it; less than full disclosure defeats the purpose of obtaining consent. If the public's need for the research is so great that it will be conducted despite the desire of potential participants not to be involved (assuming that they are fully informed), there should be a straightforward decision to that effect, not a deceitful, pro forma exercise in obtaining "informed" consent.

A second countervailing consideration concerns the competing interests of providing protection for confidential information and supplying accurate information to participants. If a researcher who desires to alert participants to the risks of disclosure constructs a consent form that confers no such promise or expectation of privacy, that researcher may inadvertently weaken his or her case in subsequent legal proceedings that seek to prove that confidentiality was respected, thus actually placing participants at a greater risk of disclosure (Gray & Melton, 1985; Melton, 1983). On the other hand, a researcher who promises participants confidentiality that is not based on any legal right may be misinforming the participants, thus failing to provide sufficient accurate information on which to base consent. Promises of confidentiality that are not based on any legal right may not be recognized and may result in liability to the researcher for voluntary breaches of such promises (Gray & Melton, 1985).

The case of *Kennedy v. Connecticut Department of Public Safety* (1987) provides an example of a researcher promising a level of confidentiality that was without legal basis but that was considered by the court as providing some protection of confidentiality. There, a candidate for her doctorate in sociology included in her informed consent form a statement that "under no circumstances will the facts observed, or the opinions held by the P.I. [Principal Investigator] be revealed to any other party" (p. 498). In this sexual discrimination case, the plaintiff (suing party) sought to discover information from this researcher, who was conducting her research at the time and place the discriminatory conduct allegedly occurred. The court held that the information sought was subject to discovery (i.e., compelled disclosure to the party filing suit). However, they did give weight to the fact that the scholar obtained certain information following a promise of confidentiality. "Requiring her on this record to divulge the identities of those individuals who communicated with her under a promise of confidentiality conceivably could needlessly jeopardize an important scholar-subject trust relationship without clearly serving a transcendent interest" (p. 501). Accordingly, she was allowed to delete from the documents that she produced (at her own expense) the names of individuals who communicated to her expecting confidentiality.

A third countervailing consideration to complete disclosure of all potential risks of a breach of confidentiality is noted in the Belmont Report (1975), which recognizes that a special problem for consent arises when informing participants of some pertinent aspect of the research is likely to impair the validity of the research. The possibility exists that disclosure of all potential breaches of confidentiality (and all other possible harm) could impair the validity of the research. Two types of effects are especially likely to occur.

First, revelations about potential breaches of confidentiality may affect disproportionately or systematically potential participants in ways that result in biased group samples (e.g., Lidz & Roth, 1983). For example, if prospective participants in a project involving HIV testing were informed that the disclosure of test results with identifying information was legally compelled and that there were several potential risks of such disclosures (e.g., further disclosures to insurance companies, etc.), it seems likely that potential participants who considered themselves at high risk for HIV infection would be less likely to agree to participate than would those who had little reason to believe that they would test positively. The result would be that a sample that was assumed to be random was, in fact, biased. The biased selection would lead to results of highly questionable validity.

Response bias is a second potential problem in research data analysis that flows from the disclosure of risks of a breach of confidentiality. Singer (1978) reported support for the hypothesis that absolute confidentiality enhances both the rate and quality of responses to sensitive questions. Thus, persons who, because of their belief that absolute confidentiality will be maintained, agree to participate in research may respond more than those persons who agree but have no such guarantee that responses will be confidential. If such a response bias (a) was particularly likely to occur in a particular research project and (b) would compromise seriously the integrity of the findings, the researcher may have grounds for a less than complete disclosure of potential risks.

Most questions in AIDS-related research are quite sensitive and, thus, are likely to result in similar effects. This conclusion, however, is far from clear. Turner (1982), for example, provided evidence that verbalized guarantees of confidentiality are met with respondent skepticism and outright disbelief. Similarly, Singer (1983) offered several reasons for minimal effects on responses from informed consent procedures.

The ethical guidelines outlined in the Belmont Report (1975) for research involving incomplete disclosure state that such research is justified only if it is clear that (a) incomplete disclosure is truly necessary to accomplish the goals of the research; (b) there are no undisclosed risks to participants that are more than minimal; and (c) there is an adequate plan for debriefing participants and for dissemination of research results to them, when appropriate. Furthermore, the report recommends that information about risks should never be withheld for the purpose of eliciting cooperation of participants and that truthful answers should always be given to direct questions about the research. Care should be taken to distinguish cases in which disclosure would destroy or invalidate the research from those in which disclosure would simply inconvenience the investigator.

Department of Health and Human Services regulations (Protection of Human Subjects, 45 C.F.R. § 46.116[d], 1992 [Health and Human Services]); see also § 116[c]) relating to incomplete disclosures state that:

> (d) An IRB may approve a consent procedure which does not include, or which alters, some or all of the elements of informed consent set forth in this section, or waive the requirements to obtain informed consent provided the IRB finds and documents that:
> (1) The research involves no more than minimal risk to the subjects;
> (2) The waiver or alteration will not adversely affect the rights and welfare of the subjects;

(3) The research could not practicably be carried out without the waiver or alteration; and

(4) Whenever appropriate, the subjects will be provided with additional pertinent information after participation.

Despite this provision for an alteration of consent requirements, it seems unlikely that withholding potential risks of a breach of confidentiality and the consequent harmful effects would be approved. It would be difficult to argue that withholding information concerning potential risks from an unauthorized disclosure would not affect adversely the welfare of the participants or that it would involve no more than minimal risk. Additionally, unlike some deception in research that may be explained during debriefing, it would be difficult to convince participants after the data were collected that the research could not have been conducted without a full disclosure of risks. The participants so misled might demand to have their data destroyed at that time, presumably before it could be analyzed. Given participants' legal and ethical right to withdraw from the research at any time, the researchers would have to comply with such requests.

The FDA regulations differ from DHHS in this section. The FDA does not provide for the authority to waive this requirement, except in cases of emergency (21 C.F.R. § 50.23, 1993).

Description of Benefits

In addition to disclosure of potential risks and harm, researchers, pursuant to the third informed consent rule of the DHHS, must also provide a description of any benefits participants may reasonably expect from the research (Protection of Human Subjects, 45 C.F.R. § 46.116[a][2]–[3], 1992 [Health and Human Services]). Because it has been "too late" for most AIDS research participants to benefit directly from their participation, beneficence toward others is often a major inducement. Researchers in this context carry a special burden to ensure that their studies are designed well and are likely to produce those benefits (e.g., Novick, 1990a).

The potential benefit of research also may be difficult to gauge, because serendipitous findings may be the ones that have the most impact. It should be possible, however, to give participants a general sense of what the investigator hopes to accomplish through the research (e.g., to learn more about how stress and the immune system are related) and any easily identifiable benefits, such as payment for participation.

If, as a result of their involvement, participants will be deprived of benefits, this point should be made clear. In particular, research on the efficacy of specific preventive or therapeutic interventions may necessitate at least temporary deprivation of other interventions (e.g., Breger, 1983; McLean, 1980). When such withholding of services is part of the research design, sufficient information about the risks and benefits of those services must also be given to permit potential participants to make an informed decision.

Description of Alternative Procedures

The fourth informed consent requirement becomes increasingly important for AIDS research as experimental drug trials continue to increase. This requirement states that "there must be disclosure of appropriate alternative procedures or courses of treatment, if any, that might be advantageous to the subject" (§ 46.116[a][4]).

For example, assume that investigators plan to test a new "therapeutic" drug that is hoped to be more effective than AZT in retarding the progression of the disease but that has unknown long-term effects. According to this requirement, the researchers would have to disclose to potential participants in the informed consent process the potential benefits of AZT and any other treatment that might be advantageous, in addition to those of the drug being tested.

Description of Measures to Assure Confidentiality

Investigators are also required to inform potential participants about the procedures for maintaining confidentiality and the limits on privacy: "There must be a statement describing the extent, if any, to which confidentiality of records identifying the subject will be maintained" (§ 46.116[a][5]).

Compliance with this requirement mandates that AIDS researchers be at once candid as to potential breaches of confidentiality and firm in their commitment to confidentiality and measures to ensure it (Bayer, Levine & Murray, 1984; Gray & Melton, 1985). Only when prospective participants have been informed about possible harm that may result from breaches of confidentiality may they calculate the likelihood that such harm will materialize. Unfortunately, some researchers have concerned themselves much too little with those threats to confidentiality that ensue after the study is completed. Such disregard for potential breaches of confidentiality has serious ramifications in AIDS research, where disclosures can be devastating to the participants.

The Revised Code of Ethics of the American Sociological Association (1982, p. 10) addresses post hoc threats to confidentiality directly in requiring that "confidential information provided by research participants must be treated as such by sociologists, even when this information enjoys no legal protection or privilege and legal force is applied." Full disclosure of the limits of confidentiality protects both the participant and the researcher. A claim of misrepresentation can be made against researchers who promise absolute confidentiality when they are aware of the possibility that a court order may compel disclosure.

It is clear that, under the current law, absolute guarantees of confidentiality cannot be offered. Participants should be informed whether information will be retained after the research is completed and, if so, (a) for how long, (b) in what form, and (c) with what safeguards. Perhaps most important, all reasonably foreseeable breaches of confidentiality should be explained to participants.

The point at which a particular probability rises to the level of "reasonably foreseeable" is, of course, a matter of judgment. Some guidance is offered, however, by the overarching principle of respect due to participants. That standard suggests that investigators should err on the side of overinclusiveness in describing risks. Certainly, the possibility of subpoenas should be acknowledged, absent clear sources of legal protection, such as a privilege statute (see, e.g., Gray & Melton, 1985, and Chap. 5).

Types of Disclosure

As discussed in more detail in Chapter 3, there are four broad categories of data disclosure. First, there are disclosures that involve minimal risk to the privacy of participants and may occur without consent or further notice. Examples of this type of disclosure include the release of unidentified, summarized information disclosed to other researchers through publication. Because these disclosures do not place participants at risk, consent is not required.

Second, disclosures may be made that *do* involve significant threats to privacy but do not require the consent of participants. Examples of this type of disclosure include the release of information pursuant to subpoenas or other legal process (e.g., search warrant). Because the researcher may not withhold the information that is being sought, consent neither is required nor relevant.

The third category of disclosure involves those that require consent but to which participants consented as a condition of participation in the study. Under this scheme, in deciding to consent to the study, the participant agrees to any such subsequent disclosures. An example of this type of disclosure is provided by FDA regulations.

The fourth type of disclosure includes those that require the consent of participants but for which consent was not obtained initially. In such circumstances, participants obviously must be contacted again. In these cases they must have already consented to the maintenance of identifying information and future intrusions by the researcher. This latter type of consent is frequently provided in connection with longitudinal studies wherein participants may be contacted repeatedly over the course of an extensive period of time.

The detailed descriptions by researchers of reasonably foreseeable potential confidentiality disclosures provide participants with a forewarning of possible harm resulting from disclosures, even though they may not be avoidable. Thus forewarned, potential research participants (and/or substitute decision makers) can decide for themselves whether to become involved in the research and risk the harm flowing from breaches of confidentiality. Recall, however, that informed consent does not require disclosure of information regarding *all* potential harm, however remote (e.g., Description of Harmful Effects subsection of the Required Disclosures section above).

The Lambda Legal Defense and Education Fund (1984, pp. 27–29) has provided a guide that recommends the following steps to protect the confidentiality of data:

1. Researchers should not collect identifying information if it is not necessary.
2. If there is a need for identifying information, participants should be informed beforehand as to what identifying information may or may not be treated confidentially.
3. Researchers should enter into an agreement clearly specifying that the information will not be released to third parties without participants' written consent and that the information will be used only by those working on that particular research project.
4. Researchers should guarantee that if they receive a subpoena or similar order, they will notify participants of same and will make every effort to resist such orders.
5. Researchers who are given permission to disseminate identifying information to third parties should be required to bind those third

parties to the same strict standards of confidentiality to which the researchers are held.

6. Any possible risks associated with the disclosure of identifying information should be explained to the subject prior to participation in the research program.

7. To avoid the inadvertent release of identifying information, internal procedures and safeguards should be developed to separate identifying information from nonidentifying information so that the former is disclosed only in connection with essential uses in the research.

8. All researchers, researchers' assistants, and all others connected with the project should provide these guarantees.

(See the Office for Protection from Research Risks (OPRR), National Institutes of Health (NIH), 1984, pp. 1–5, for similar recommendations.)

Compensation for Injury

In addition to alerting potential research participants of possible confidentiality disclosures, it is very important in AIDS research to inform potential participants about remedies that will be available if participants are harmed as a result of their involvement in research. For research involving more than minimal risk, there must be an explanation of any compensation or medical treatments that are available if injury occurs and what they consist of or where further information may be obtained (45 C.F.R. § 46.116[a][6]). For all research, investigators must disclose whom to contact for answers to questions about the research itself, the rights of participants, and research-related injuries (45 C.F.R. § 46.116[a][7]).

"Minimal risk" exists when "the risks of harm anticipated in the proposed research are not greater, considering probability and magnitude, than those ordinarily encountered in daily life or during the performance of routine physical or psychological examinations or tests" (45 C.F.R. § 46.102[g]) and, "that the probability and magnitude of harm or discomfort anticipated in the research are not greater in and of themselves than those ordinarily encountered in daily life or during the performance of routine physical or psychological examinations or tests" (e.g., Protection of Human Subjects, 45 C.F.R. 690.102[i], 1992 [National Science Foundation]).

Although the regulations leave room for omission of compensation for research-induced injuries (provided that disclosure is made that compensation may be omitted), it is questionable whether such a position is ethically defensible, especially when the research clearly was not for the benefit of the participants. If people give of themselves, compensation for, or free treatment of, injuries incurred as a result seems to be a minimal expectation so that participants are not subjected to de facto punishment for their altruism. Even when participants may expect to benefit directly (as in treatment research), the likelihood is that they are risking receipt of "treatment" (e.g., placebos) known to be ineffective or agreeing to forego treatments that have at least some documented efficacy (e.g., AZT). Accordingly, compensation or treatment for injuries still seems to be a minimal expectation.

In AIDS research, such expectations are likely to arise in two contexts. First, in intervention research, when participants are subjected to iatrogenic effects (negative side effects) or are deprived of treatments or preventive measures known to have at least some positive effects, researchers arguably bear a duty to provide treatment to remediate any untoward effects. For example, in many such studies some participants receive the treatment drug, others receive a placebo, and the study is conducted blindly so that the participants are unaware of who is receiving the treatment drug and who is receiving the placebo. In this situation, the participants are likely to experience anxiety because they are hoping to receive the treatment drug and, in fact, may be involved in such research for the purpose of obtaining treatment.

Second, when research procedures themselves create psychological or social harm, researchers ought to make treatment easily available. For example, the need for counseling is likely in AIDS research. If a participant is tested for HIV and the results are positive, the researcher must expect to provide or arrange for extensive support while such information is being disclosed and after such disclosure is made. Individuals who already experience ambivalence or anxiety concerning their sexuality may experience panic when responding to survey items relating to sexual orientation. Moreover, questionnaire items may inadvertently confirm those myths held by research participants.

It should be noted, however, that the Ethical Principles of Psychologists (APA, 1992) do not expressly require researchers to take any remedial action. Rather, the Ethical Principles, like the federal regulations, merely require that potential participants be informed about material information (i.e., "significant factors that may be expected to influence their willingness to participate"; Std. 6.11[b]), presumably but not expressly including whether compensation or treatment will be available if harm is experienced and, if so, whether there are any limitations on the kind or amount available. The absence of an express requirement in the Principles is one of the ways that the elements of disclosure promulgated by the Principles vary from those specified in the federal regulations. Note, however, that the Principles do require researchers to clarify services to be offered as *inducements* (as distinguished from *compensation* or *treatment* for research-induced injuries) for participation in research (Std. 6.14[a]).

Regardless of the absence of an express provision to that effect, a duty to rectify harm in research can be reasonably inferred from the general principles of beneficence and nonmaleficence (APA, 1992, Preamble and Prin. E) and the specific duty to avoid or minimize harm (Std. 1.14). Such a duty may also be implicit in the duty of researchers to "honor all commitments that they have made to research participants" (Std. 6.19), because such commitments may reasonably be expected by participants knowledgeable about the roles of clinical researchers. Presumably though, such an expectation could be abrogated through an express disclosure that compensation or treatment for research-induced injuries will not be provided.

In that regard, the drafters of both the federal regulations and the Ethical Principles may have recognized both an implicit social contract and the practical limitations on investigators' ability to fulfill it. Thus, an express waiver may avoid a breach of implicit promises and leave prospective participants to decide whether they are motivated sufficiently to suffer a triple loss—their time, the harm, and the absence of compensation or treatment for the harm—to contribute to knowledge.

Voluntariness

Finally, potential participants should be assured of the voluntary nature of their participation in the research and of their right to make an informed decision. "There should be a statement that participation is voluntary, refusal to participate will involve no penalty of loss of benefits to which the participants are otherwise entitled, and that the participants may discontinue participation at any time without penalty or loss of benefits to which they are otherwise entitled" (§ 46.116[a][8]).

The Belmont Report (1975) stressed that research participation requires conditions free of coercion and undue influence. The report described coercion as occurring when an overt threat of harm is presented intentionally by one person to another to obtain compliance. In contrast, the Report defined undue influence as occurring through the offer of an excessive, unwarranted, inappropriate, or improper reward or other overture to obtain compliance. Further, the report noted that inducements that ordinarily would be acceptable may become undue influences if the participant is especially vulnerable.

To be sure, research participants with fatal illnesses are vulnerable in many ways. Therefore, AIDS researchers must be especially careful to ensure that inducements offered for research participation are not effectively coercive (see APA, 1992, Std. 6.14). Participants may deny the significance of their diseases or, conversely, deny the risks of treatment—all from desperation. The Belmont Report recognized that a continuum of influencing factors exists and that it is impossible to state precisely where justifiable persuasion ends and undue influence begins. Nevertheless, AIDS researchers should strive to make such distinctions.

The identification and explanation of extant influencing factors at the onset of participation in research, while important, are potentially insufficient. AIDS researchers must also ensure that significant new findings developed during the course of the research are provided to participants in a timely manner—at least inasmuch as those findings might reasonably be expected to affect participants' willingness to continue in the project (e.g., indications that the new "treatment drug" being tested may cause serious side effects for some people). Also it is worth noting that the consent process may not be used to obtain waivers of participants' rights in the event that the investigator or research institution incurs liability (45 C.F.R. § 46.116; OPRR at 2).

Procedures for Obtaining Informed Consent

In addition to attending to *what* participants will be consenting to (i.e., which factors are included in the consent form), AIDS researchers need to consider both *how* such informed consent is obtained and from *whom*. Investigators, granting agencies, and IRBs should give careful thought to the procedures for obtaining informed consent, as well as the substance of what is disclosed.

AIDS researchers should be aware that written forms are not necessarily the optimal means of providing information (particularly for children) or of documenting consent. Obviously, written forms provide a largely indisputable record of the consent and, in doing so, provide some legal protection to the researcher. However, there are two considerations that should discourage excessive or exclusive reliance on written forms.

The Consent Form: Countervailing Considerations

Participants often do not comprehend or attend carefully to written forms (Lidz, 1984). In view of the significance of the decision to be made, the researcher bears a special obligation to ensure that consent is truly informed. If written forms are used, special attention should be given to their readability, taking into consideration the level of reading comprehension of potential participants (Elwork, Sales & Alfini, 1982; Grundner, 1978). The written forms should be supplemented by discussion (Roth et al., 1982), and consideration should be given to the use of two-part consent forms. A two-part consent form includes questions at the end to ensure that prospective participants understand the information that has been disclosed. Stanley (1987) has provided an excellent discussion of the comprehension of informed consent forms.

Because of the nature of AIDS, concern for prospective participants' comprehension of information conveyed through informed consent procedures is heightened. The complexity of AIDS often requires that considerable information regarding symptoms be presented in detail (i.e., because AIDS results in vulnerability to countless opportunistic infections, explanations of side effects of withholding AZT, for example, necessarily will be lengthy). Moreover, because AIDS often involves degradation of mental processes, the ability to give competent consent may be compromised.

An issue in the allocation of authority for decisions about research participation of AIDS patients who have become incompetent is that their preference for substitute decision makers (if expressed when competent) may be different from the "natural" choice that the law and clinicians may recognize, absent an express advance directive by the patient (Nelson, 1989). Only one-third of gay men with AIDS identify legally recognized relatives as their preferred surrogate decision makers (Steinbrook et al., 1986).

Not only do consent forms potentially fail to provide comprehensible information to prospective participants but also such forms themselves may pose a threat to the confidentiality of participants. If identifying information is removed from research data, the forms may represent the only identifiable record of a particular participant's involvement in a study. The mere existence of the forms, thus, leaves participants vulnerable to disclosures through subpoenas or other inquiries. It is worth remembering that private behavior may be inferred—inaccurate as those inferences may be—from the nature of the study. The use and retention of consent forms would be unwise when anonymous surveys are conducted on the street (e.g., outside bathhouses) or with groups of stigmatized individuals (e.g., associations of gay men; clients in drug treatment programs or runaway shelters) about private or illegal behavior and attitudes. When consent forms do present a demonstrable threat to privacy, federal regulations permit consent without such documentation; DHHS regulations, for example, state that:

(c) an IRB may waive the requirement for the investigator to obtain a signed consent form for some or all subjects if it finds either:

(1) that the only record linking the subject and the research would be the consent document and the principal risk would be potential harm resulting from a breach of confidentiality. Each subject will be asked whether the subject wants documentation linking the subject with the research, and the subject's wishes will govern, or

(2) that the research presents no more than minimal risk of harm to subjects and involves no procedures for which written consent is normally required outside of the research context. (45 C.F.R. § 46.117[c])

In cases where the documentation requirement is waived, the IRB may require the investigator to provide subjects with a written statement regarding the research. Current FDA regulations also provide for an IRB waiver of the requirement for signed consent when the principal risk is a breach of confidentiality. Examples of this kind of research relevant to AIDS include epidemiological studies and other surveys. Like DHHS regulations, current FDA regulations allow for an IRB waiver of documentation of informed consent in instances of minimal risk.

FDA regulations permit the use of either a written consent document that embodies the elements of informed consent or a "short form" stating that the elements of informed consent have been presented orally to participants. When this form is used, there must be a witness to the oral presentation and IRB review and approval of a written summary of the information presented to participants. Participants or their legally authorized representatives, if necessary, must sign the short form. The witness must sign both the short form and a copy of the summary, and the person obtaining the consent must sign a copy of the summary. Participants or their representatives must be given a copy of the summary as well as a copy of the short form.

Competency

In addition to providing for confidential and other procedures for obtaining informed consent and structuring a consent form in such a way that all relevant information is presented to participants in an understandable manner, AIDS researchers must determine from whom consent, and assent, should and/or must be obtained and how this determination should be made. These concerns are applicable to AIDS research surprisingly (and unfortunately) often. Examples of circumstances in which these issues arise include sex surveys of adolescents and behavioral surveys of runaways. The Code of Federal Regulations contains additional provisions for the protection of children involved as participants in research (45 C.F.R. § 46.401–9). "Children" are defined as "persons who have not attained the legal age for consent to treatments or procedures involved in the research, under the applicable law of the jurisdiction in which the research will be conducted" (45 C.F.R. § 46.412[a]).

Unfortunately, this definition does not help to clarify applicable standards for research when state laws are in conflict with federal regulations. In general, when state law demands a higher standard than federal law, federal law does not preempt state law. Thus, although federal regulations may require that assent be obtained from children seven years of age or older, if state law requires assent from children age five or above, state law would be the appropriate standard to follow. The age at which parental permission is required is equally unclear when state law conflicts with federal regulations. In any event, one *cannot* assume that legislatures that lower the age of majority for consent to treatment of a particular condition would also do so for consent to research related to that condition (see Areen, 1992). Legislators might desire, for example, to ensure that treatment is available to minors who would not receive it if they were not able to seek treatment on their own (note that the legislators' motive is protection of child welfare, not child autonomy and privacy), but they also may wish to ensure that children are provided special protection from risky research. Usually, there are neither statutes nor cases on which to rely for the answer.

Generally, potential participants who have not reached the age of majority are not legally capable of consenting to participation in research. Consequently, a parent or legal guardian must give permission for children to participate in research (e.g., § 46.408[b]). However, there are exceptions to this requirement. Thus, persons who have reached the age of majority are able to give consent to participation (if not incompetent on other grounds), as are some potential participants who have not reached the legally defined age of majority (§ 46.408[c]).

Grisso (1992) described the circumstances under which § 46.408[c] allows minors' participation in research without prior consent from the children's parents or guardians. He explained, for example, that if the IRB determines that a research protocol applies to conditions or a participant population for which parental or guardian permission is not a reasonable requirement for the protection of participants (e.g., neglected or abused children), then it may waive the DHHS requirements for informed consent and parental permission as long as an appropriate mechanism for protecting minor research participants is substituted, and waiver is not inconsistent with federal, state, or local law.

Grisso (1992) commented on four situations that might justify a waiver of the requirement for parental or guardian permission suggested by the National Commission for the Protection of Human Subjects in Biomedical and Behavioral Research (1977). Grisso also noted that, contrary to the commission's suggestion, it is difficult to imagine situations in which parental incompetence or intellectual deficiency would constitute adequate justification for waiver of the requirement for parental or guardian permission under 46.408(c)—at least for most social science and behavioral research proposals. Where there has been a formal declaration of incompetence of the parent, society usually will have authorized a guardian who can provide the required permission. And where there has been no declaration of parental incompetence, parents arguably retain independent interests that should be included in decisions regarding their child's research participation. He argued that their incapacities suggest the need for additional protections for the child, but need not include resorting to circumvention of parental authority. This argument seems to carry greatest weight when the parents at issue are minimally incompetent and "loving." Although this is surely the case much of the time, parents' interests in their children's participation may well be disinterested or self-serving.

However true Grisso's arguments may be generally, the etiology and epidemiology of AIDS magnify issues of parental competence and availability. HIV's tropism for brain cells, coupled with the sudden onset of AIDS-related disorders, may result in a parent being rendered incompetent or unavailable long before legal systems can respond (e.g., Michaels & Levine, 1992). Therefore, it is not difficult to imagine cases wherein parental incompetence or intellectual deficiency would constitute adequate justification for waiving parental permission requirements. For example, drug-abusing parents with AIDS-related dementia in its late stages are not more competent to make decisions about experimental treatments or vaccines merely because they have not been formally declared incompetent than are those similarly situated individuals who have formally been declared incompetent. Perhaps a middle ground—protecting both parental autonomy and children's welfare—has been reached by New York's new statute providing for appointment of standby guardians whom parents (before their becoming incompetent) may designate to assume their parental responsibilities when the parents die, when they are certified as incompetent by their physician, or when they consent to the appointment (1992 N.Y. Sess. Law News ch. 290 [A. 10966-A][McKinney]).

The parental incompetence exception applies when parents are physically present but lack the requisite mental capacity to give informed consent. The next exception applies when parents, for whatever reason, are physically uninvolved in their children's lives. Grisso (1992) observed that this type of situation generally occurs when the behavioral research at issue involves an aspect of the minors' lives over which the law has given them control without parental involvement. For example, many states have provisions whereby minors may seek treatment without parental consent (e.g., sexually transmitted diseases, suicidal ideation, drug abuse). Because minors in those circumstances are legally capable of consenting to treatment on their own, parental consent is not required.

A third situation justifying reliance on minors' sole consent to research participation arises when the parents are competent and available but their orientation toward their children is not beneficent. Grisso (1992) noted that such a situation generally is the result of a breakdown in the parent-child relationship to the extent that it cannot be assumed that parents will act benevolently to protect their children's interest when deciding whether to participate in research (e.g., abuse/neglect situations). This same problem may occur when consent is sought from guardians, in that the guardians' interests may create pressure for minors to agree to research requests when such acquiescence is not in their best interest. Thus, there are circumstances for which requiring the permission of parents or of authorized guardians may actually work against the principle of affording protection for minors' autonomous assent. Situations such as these raise the possibility that parental or guardian permission is not a reasonable requirement to protect the minor's interests.

Finally, the commission suggests that when parents are competent, available, and beneficent, but their participation is superfluous, minors should be allowed to give authoritative consent to research participation. Grisso (1992) observed that this type of situation is generally relevant when the minor is a "mature minor" (e.g., emancipated). However, Grisso has stated that parental permission is not rendered unreasonable in all cases merely because the minors do not seem to need protection. Although a number of reviews of empirical research and theory suggest that adolescents' capacities to understand, reason, and make voluntary decisions in informed consent procedures are not significantly different from those of adults (e.g., Melton, Koocher & Saks, 1983; Weithorn, 1983), Grisso noted that there is likely to be considerable heterogeneity among adolescents with regard to these abilities. This, he suggested, means that for some proportion of prospective adolescent participants these abilities are poorly developed, even as compared with the "average" adolescent. Grisso has also observed that none of the relevant research has been conducted with adolescents in stressful circumstances. Stress, which is likely to be a factor in AIDS research, Grisso argued, may impair functioning in these domains.

Additional Safeguards When Minors Themselves Consent

Grisso (1992) stated his agreement with the implicit assumption of DHHS regulations that additional precautionary measures are necessary to protect minors whenever parents or guardians are not involved directly in the consent process. Whatever these measures are, they should ensure several things: first, that the minors clearly understand the proposed procedures and their purposes; second, that they be in a position to make an autonomous decision to assent or refuse, relatively free from conditions that might cause them to "volunteer" against their will; and third, that they possess similar autonomy with regard to discontinuation of participation, if that desire should arise. Section 46.408(c) offers several considerations: the nature of the procedures that participants will undergo, the risks and benefits, and the age, maturity, status, and conditions of the minors themselves.

The Permission/Denial and Assent/Refusal Dichotomies

The considerations for and against providing special protection to minors in situations where adult permission is not required are similar to the issues raised in assessing the competency of minors for consent and assent more generally. In addition to minors' right to consent to research participation without parental consent in some situations, they generally are given the right to assent or decline to participitate in research. Grisso (1992) explained DHHS Federal Regulation 46.408(b) as establishing the parents' prerogative of "permitting" or "denying" their child's participation. "Denial" blocks the child's participation. But "permission," unlike "consent," does not mandate automatically the child's participation. Section 46.408(a) gives the minor the authority to decide to "assent" or "refuse." Thus, the minor's research participation ordinarily can occur only when parental and child permission coalesce. Either a parent's denial of permission or a child's refusal precludes the child's participation.

According to the Code of Federal Regulations, the acting IRB shall determine that adequate provisions have been made for soliciting the assent of the children when, in the judgment of the IRB, the children are capable of providing assent. "Assent" is defined as "a child's affirmative agreement to participate in research. Mere failure to object should not, absent affirmative agreement, be construed as assent" (§ 46.402[b]).

DHHS requirements for assent state: "In determining whether children are capable of assenting, the IRB shall take into account the ages, maturity, and psychological state of the children involved. This judgment may be made for all children to be involved in research under a particular protocol, or for each child, as the IRB deems appropriate" ("Additional Protections for Children," 45 C.F.R. § 46.408[a], 1993).

Although the research guidelines of the Department of Health, Education, and Welfare (1973; DHEW, now DHHS) required that assent be obtained from children seven years of age or older, the issue of the age of minors as it relates to actual competency is far from resolved. A study by Keith-Spiegel (1983) conducted some years ago is illustrative. In that study, a consent survey was sent to authorities in child development areas asking them to specify the age at which minors generally are as capable as adults of meaningfully assenting to participation in a study, the description of which was fairly straightforward. Their answers ranged from 2 to 17, with a mean age of 11.

The foregoing analysis suggests that legal establishment of a particular age at which minors are capable of assent or consent would not be especially helpful. Rather, researchers need a method of developmentally assessing the capacity of minors to agree to participate (assuming, of course, the minors are given developmentally appropriate information) (Keith-Spiegel, 1983). In 1977 the National Commission for the Protection of Human Subjects of Biomedical and Behavioral Science Research issued a report entitled "Research Involving Children." Although this report comprised one of the most thorough and definitive considerations of issues surrounding competency to consent and is fraught with references to the wishes of minor participants, the report does not address methods of assessing their competence (Keith-Spiegel, 1983).

Researchers interested in exploring methods of assessing the capacities of minors to consent and assent are urged to consult works by Roth, Meisel, and Lidz (1977) and Stanley (1987) for information relating to five functional tests of competency. Grisso (1992) offered a description of a pilot assent study that can be employed for judging adolescents' capacities to consent to participation in research projects. He observed that "researchers can and should be much more creative in developing ways to demonstrate empirically that the informing process in assent procedures with minors has achieved its intended purpose" (p. 125). Such procedures are valuable tools for refining assent forms and procedures in ways that increase participants' understanding of the presented information.

It has been asserted elsewhere (Tapp & Melton, 1983) that the focus on assessing competency is misplaced. Instead of asking whether a child *is* competent to assent, one should ask whether a child *could be taught* to exercise competent decision making. Whether this obligation should be required ethically of researchers is yet to be decided. Certainly it is not required legally. It is, however, legally required that researchers determine who is competent to assent to research (difficult as this may be) and obtain such assent in addition to acquiring consent from legally authorized adults, when required.

There are exceptions that provide for bypassing children's decision making (allowing a waiver of the minor's assent) in two circumstances: in research that is very important for the health or well-being of the child or when "they cannot reasonably be consulted" due to serious impairment impinging on competency (e.g., severely impaired intellectual capacities). When assent is not received from a child participant, the importance of "proxy consent" of course is heightened.

According to DHHS's requirements, "If the IRB determines that the capability of some or all of the children is so limited that they cannot reasonably be consulted or that the intervention or procedure involved in the research holds out a prospect of direct benefit that is important to the health or well-being of the children and is available only in the context of the research, the assent of the children is not a necessary condition for proceeding with the research" (§ 46.408[a]). The policy concerns underlying this provision are similar to those underlying provisions relating to additional protection in research involving fetuses and pregnant women, who may also be involved in AIDS research of many types ("Additional Protections Pertaining to Research," 45 C.F.R. § 46.201, 1992). Thus, if there are minimal risks involved in the research or if there is potential for significant benefit to the child or fetus, the parents may give their consent for participation in the absence of assent by the participant.

Special Considerations

Relatively greater potential harm or relatively decreased potential benefits involved in research may require the permission of both parents (if living and entitled to custody) rather than the consent of only one (§ 46.408[b]). Obtaining permission for children who are wards of the state to participate in research may be even more difficult (§ 46.409). With the increased incidence of foster care for children with AIDS, research permission requirements from state agencies may inhibit research with this population.

Children who are wards of the state or any other agency, institution, or entity can be included in research conducted or supported by DHHS only if such research is "(1) related to their status as wards; or (2) conducted in schools, camps, hospitals, institutions, or similar settings in which the majority of children involved as subjects are not wards" (§ 46.409[a]). If researchers include child participants who are wards of the state and their participation requires any type of travel arrangements or other inconveniences to those persons responsible for them (e.g., foster parents), researchers also should seek assent from these persons, although such assent is not required by regulation.

Even if the previously described consent problems are resolved in a particular case at the onset of research, problems may arise in ongoing research when legal guardianship changes or when an individual's mental ability declines as a result of the progression of AIDS (e.g., AIDS dementia), leaving the individual incompetent to utilize her or his right to terminate participation in research. For example, if the legal guardian of a child with AIDS has consented to research that includes ongoing testing for six months but then loses guardianship during this period, must the new guardian also give permission or assent to the research? Must assent from participants be obtained more than once during a longitudinal study in anticipation of the possibility that the person, at some time during the research, becomes incapable of consenting to such research? Unfortunately, commentary on such issues is scarce.

Conclusion

The sheer magnitude of the ethical implications suggests that they will not be dismissed easily. Informed consent formalities are a necessary but not sufficient means of safeguarding the interests of participants. Informed consent procedures must necessarily go beyond mere formalities if those interests are to be protected adequately. This chapter provides what must be characterized as only a first step toward that end—an introduction to the issues at stake and the particular legal means of protecting them.

Chapter 3

LEGALLY SANCTIONED ENCROACHMENTS ON CONFIDENTIALITY

Our society in general and our legal system in particular may be fairly characterized as being engaged in constant struggles to achieve balance. Indeed, our legal system may be viewed as a seemingly endless series of interrelated fulcrums on which are balancing apparently infinite interests. When Robert Gallo made his "discovery," he sought the protection of the patent statutes. Those statutes, which are designed to further developments in research and technology, are crafted carefully to strike a balance among competing interests that will benefit research maximally. If the patent scope and length are too small, researchers may not have sufficient incentive to invest precious resources into research. On the other hand, if the scope and temporal limitations are too expansive, research efforts may be impaired by the retention of new technologies in the hands of too few.

The body of patent law is a particular example of laws regulating competition. Antitrust law provides a framework wherein competition can flourish. Laws against unfair competition, on the other hand, provide a framework wherein competition is constrained. Examples of this kind of symbiosis abound in the law. It is an important conceptual framework for researchers to apprehend before embarking on a more thorough exploration of the manner in which competing interests are balanced.

The dangers faced by researchers attempting to weigh these interests on their own are twofold. First, researchers may not be aware of the interests that militate against affording protection at various stages throughout the research process. Second, researchers may weigh the research interests in ways that differ from the courts. Whether this is the product of researchers overvaluing their particular research or courts undervaluing it, the result is the same: a misapprehension of what the courts will do in a particular instance. The disparity between what researchers believe courts ought to do and what the courts actually do is certainly understandable, but that does not obviate the need to look beyond one's own perspective in attempting to assess accurately how one's own interests will be balanced against the interests of others.

Several principles underlie the notion of confidentiality. One of these principles requires that we respect the implied or express wishes of the person providing the information that it not be disseminated. It is also widely believed that at least some of the information provided would not be made available were it not for the expectation that it would be held in confidence. A number of other principles may operate, depending on the context of the confidential communications. In short, typically, there are a great many reasons to respect confidentiality.

Although there are often competing interests, it is clear that the forced disclosure of identifiable data in AIDS research may result in substantial costs for participants, researchers, and society. Therefore, it is important to examine carefully the ways in which disclosure may be compelled legally or not prohibited legally. Such scrutiny may help investigators to foresee and, when possible, prevent unplanned disclosures. It may also enable policy makers to identify the need to strengthen legal protection of the confidentiality of data gathered in research on AIDS (Bayer, Levine & Murray, 1984). Study of potential requirements for involuntary disclosure of data is also necessary so that researchers can accurately inform prospective participants of the limits of confidentiality.

The legal system may compel breaches of confidence in several ways. First, disclosure of records may be required or allowed pursuant to the subpoena powers of the judicial, legislative, or executive branches of state or federal government. Second, federal statutes, such as the Freedom of Information Act, may create means by which confidential information can be accessed. Third, judicially created duties may require disclosure of confidential information (see, e.g., *Tarasoff v. Regents of University of California*, 1976; and Chap. 4). Similarly, health and safety laws that mandate the reporting of AIDS, ARC, and HIV status, as well as those that stipulate the mandatory reporting of child abuse and neglect, also compromise confidentiality. Additionally, administrative regulations promulgated by governmental agencies may require release of confidential material. Finally, some "voluntary disclosures" may aptly be characterized as breaches of confidentiality. The legal system may indirectly contribute to researchers' inappropriate voluntary disclosure of research participants' confidential information by not providing proper sanctions against such disclosures.

Subpoenas

Perhaps the most serious threat to confidential material is presented by the subpoena power. Subpoenas may be issued from the judiciary for use in a pending civil or criminal case, from administrative agencies to gather information for use in administrative proceedings, or from legislatures for investigatory purposes. The use of subpoenas for confidential information about research participants is becoming increasingly common. Between 1966 and 1976 at least 50 scholars were served with subpoenas ordering them to reveal the identities of sources and participants in research (in eighteen different cases). At least thirty other scientists were threatened with subpoenas. In a national survey of researchers about 8 percent reported problems of preventing disclosure of confidential information to government authorities (Nelkin, 1984). Subpoenas for research data continue to arise, usually in product liability litigation (Holder, 1993), as might occur if behavioral-epidemiological data appeared relevant to a suit alleging problems resulting from unsafe condoms, vaccines, or therapeutic drugs.

The subpoena power represents a particularly pernicious threat to the confidentiality of participants for three reasons. First, subpoenas are often unpredictable. Second, they pose a particularly high risk that AIDS research participants may become the targets of criminal investigations. Finally, once the subpoena power has been exercised, the formerly confidential information may be widely disseminated. Although none of these threats applies exclusively to research participants in AIDS studies, they combine with other factors in ways that may be especially harmful to an already suffering class of persons.

Subpoenas as Threats to Confidentiality

Because subpoenas may be issued for reasons wholly unrelated to the purpose of research, they are highly unpredictable (see, e.g., *In re Grand Jury Subpoena*, 1984). They often arise, for example, in the context of product liability cases where the plaintiff, seeking to prove that the product has caused harm, subpoenas any research that tends to show deleterious effects. It is almost impossible to accurately predict whether a particular product will be involved in litigation. Consequently, it is difficult to accurately assess the actual risks to confidentiality. If researchers cannot accurately assess such risks, they certainly cannot communicate them to research participants. Thus, consent may not be truly informed.

Many AIDS research participants have engaged in some form of illegal conduct. Although AIDS is spreading increasingly to more diverse segments of the population, society has been slow in recognizing the shift; AIDS still is associated largely with gay men and intravenous drug users. Hence, it is possible that information gathered in the course of research may be viewed by prosecutors as potentially rife with leads relating to criminal conduct. It is plausible to envision an enterprising prosecutor seeking a subpoena for the raw data in an AIDS study to assist a grand jury in an investigation of illegal drug use or sexual conduct (Kershaw & Small, 1972).

The use of information for any purpose other than that to which participants consented is an unethical affront to the dignity of participants. In addition, when research is government-sponsored and data are used for the purpose of self-incrimination, there is arguably a violation of the fifth amendment, in addition to the breach of the agreement between the investigator and the participant. Such misuse of research data is likely to chill research on AIDS. Because of the fear that data would be misused, in the early stages of the AIDS crisis some gay organizations advised against participation in research (Office of Technology Assessment, 1985).

Once subpoenaed, material enters the public domain. Forums for such entry include litigation as well as administrative and legislative hearings. Once in the public domain, there is considerable risk of extensive dissemination of confidential information. Embarrassment or other adverse consequences may follow.

To illustrate the very real threat of the subpoena to AIDS researchers, we offer for consideration the following scenarios. Although the threats they represent are quite real, these cases are purely hypothetical. The first involves the use of a judicial subpoena in a civil suit, the second involves an administrative subpoena, and the third involves a legislative subpoena. The more thorough discussion in Chapter 5 will provide some insight into how these scenarios might be resolved.

Subpoenas in Operation

Judicial Subpoena. Consider the case of a young, gay man who has AIDS. He has been receiving drug treatments with the assurance that, at the very least, they will not worsen his condition. He hopes they will provide him with many years of life that he would not otherwise enjoy. Soon after the commencement of chemotherapy, however, his condition worsens. The diminution of his life expectancy is considerable—from one year to a month or two. He files suit against the pharmaceutical manufacturer that produces the drug for misrepresentation and the pain and suffering associated with the harmful effects of the drug. The manufacturer intends to prove that the deterioration is the result of stress and is not caused by the drug. Specifically, they assert that the young man's loss of his significant other, one week after his first drug treatment, caused his deterioration.

To facilitate the defense, the manufacturer wishes to obtain information from a study conducted by a researcher on the relationship between stress and immune functioning for AIDS patients. A subpoena is obtained by the manufacturer for all of the records, documents, findings, conclusions, notes, and other information collected during the research process. The researcher moves to quash the subpoena on the grounds that (a) the research data are of a highly sensitive and potentially embarrassing nature; (b) confidentiality was promised to the research participants before data collection; and (c) the relationship between a researcher and the participants is privileged.

Administrative Subpoena. A state public health department is actively involved in the contact tracing of persons exposed to the HIV virus by sexual contact or needle sharing. They are aware that a research project involving contact tracing of participants is being conducted to evaluate various strategies directed at behavioral change. Because both projects involve similar preventive education and counseling components and because the methodology is quite costly, the health department wants to be sure that they are not duplicating efforts and that they are casting the net broadly enough to protect the public health.

In furtherance of their goal, the health department subpoenas the names of the research participants and their contacts. The researchers involved move to quash the subpoena on the grounds that (a) confidentiality for participants and their contacts was promised and that (b) violation of the promise of confidentiality would hinder the completion of their research and thereby violate their fourteenth amendment due process rights (i.e., the government cannot deprive persons of their property [the research] without due process of law [procedural safeguards]). The researchers further assert that compliance with the subpoena would have a chilling effect on future AIDS research.

Legislative Subpoena. A state legislature is considering a bill that would require mandatory HIV testing of all prison inmates. Those testing positive would be isolated from the other inmates. Prisoners of the state argue (a) that such a law would violate their rights; (b) that the procedure is medically unwarranted in light of testing limitations (e.g., latent period between HIV infection and seropositivity); and (c) that isolation of persons with HIV is contraindicated on medical grounds.

To support their last point, the inmates cite an ongoing study on HIV transmissibility. In the interest of fully investigating these arguments, the legislature issues a subpoena for all of the research data. The researcher resists the subpoena and seeks a protective order on the grounds that (a) confidentiality was promised to the participants; (b) premature disclosure of his research data would infringe upon his academic freedom; and (c) organizing his data in their current form in ways that would be meaningful to the legislature would be overly burdensome.

Each of the scenarios presented above represents a slightly different exercise of subpoena power. The parties seeking subpoenas differ (i.e., corporation, private citizens, state agency, respectively), as do the authorities to whom the request is made (i.e., judicial, administrative, legislative). Nevertheless, they represent equally powerful threats to confidential information.

The Freedom of Information Act

Although the disclosure of AIDS research data may be compelled effectively through subpoena powers, individuals may often acquire such information much more easily without resort to subpoenas. The disclosure of confidential information may be required pursuant to either federal statutes, such as the Freedom of Information Act (FOIA, 5 U.S.C. § 552[a] [1982]) or similar state laws. Nearly every state has enacted legislation with provisions similar to the FOIA (Thurman, 1973). A discussion of these state "open record" laws would be overly complex, given their lack of uniformity. Therefore, our discussion will focus primarily on the FOIA and its impact on all federally funded research. Although we are using AIDS examples to illuminate the operation of the FOIA, the sphere of the statute's operation is, of course, much broader.

Federally supported researchers are confronted with many FOIA requests for research protocols and data from ongoing research projects. At one time the sheer quantity of data gathered in a research project automatically limited such demands, but with today's computer technology this is no longer an effective constraint. For example, a request for data from a diabetes treatment study was not considered impractical, although there were an estimated 55 million documents pertaining to 1,000 patients (Nelkin, 1984). The total number of actual instances in which an agency discloses a researcher's information against his or her wishes pursuant to the FOIA is difficult to ascertain. However, requests to the National Institutes of Health (NIH) are illustrative of the increasing use of the FOIA. NIH requests increased from 300 in 1975 to 1,638 in 1979 (Nelkin, 1984). In addition to mandatory disclosures, another impact of the FOIA is the potential for altering behavior because of the fear of FOIA-mandated disclosures. Every researcher dealing with a federal agency must prepare for at least the possibility that many different audiences will gain access to the information. Moreover, funding agencies and institutional research review boards must evaluate research projects according to their particular vulnerabilities to FOIA requests (Morris, Sales & Berman, 1981).

The FOIA is a record-keeping statute which applies broadly to all agency records "held" by government agencies. It was designed to further the people's right to know the conduct of their government through the provision of access to government information. Under the FOIA, federal agencies are required to publish notices in the *Federal Register* describing their operational policies and procedures. Federal agencies must also determine which of their records have broad public interest and must make those records available for public inspection and copying. Obviously, much of AIDS research is of broad public interest.

Should "any person" file a legitimate FOIA request for such records, they are to be provided promptly. A person making a FOIA request must follow the agency's published procedures regarding the time, place, fees, and method for specifying the desired documents. An agency, in turn, must initially respond concerning its compliance decision within 10 days of the receipt of such a request. If requesters are denied access to certain documents under the exemptions, they can appeal for an administrative review. After exhausting this administrative remedy, they can bring suit in federal court for judicial review of the agency's decision.

It is important to note that requesters do not need to allege that they have any special interest in the records or that it is in the public interest for this information to be revealed under the FOIA. All that is needed is a simple request for the documents.

FOIA and AIDS Research

The first major determination for AIDS researchers to make concerning possible FOIA requests for their data is whether any of their data are considered to be an "agency record." It is only when research is conducted under "government control" that an agency record is created for purposes of the FOIA (*Forsham v. Harris*, 1980). The term "agency record" is not statutorily defined so that the matter has been left to judicial interpretation. The FOIA empowers federal courts to order an "agency" to produce "agency records improperly withheld" from an individual requesting access (§ 552a[4][B]).

The FOIA is potentially applicable to the materials of AIDS researchers ("agency records") at almost every stage of their research (e.g., the grant or contract research proposal, reports to granting or contractual agencies, raw data, results of preliminary analyses, or final reports). The first situation in which researchers may confront the FOIA occurs when they submit a research proposal for a governmental contract or grant. The act of submitting a proposal, even if it is subsequently not awarded or funded, creates an "agency record" for FOIA purposes (*Washington Research Project v. Department of Health, Education, and Welfare*, 1974). Thus, all parts of the research proposal (e.g., the research rationale and hypotheses, the design, operationalizations of independent and dependent variables, sampling techniques, and any scales that may have been developed in the pilot work) are available to anyone upon request.

There are several dangers involved in FOIA requests for research proposals. For example, in extreme cases, an unscrupulous colleague could steal a researcher's "breakthrough" theories or methods, or the press could misinform the public about controversial hypotheses and plans for research or poison the participant pool by making potential participants aware of research hypotheses. However, such disclosure availability is not without benefits; it allows prospective grant submitters to obtain copies of proposals that have already been funded, so that they may determine the kinds of projects being funded. Moreover, some researchers take advantage of the availability of the proposals to learn how to improve their grant-writing ability (Morris et al., 1981).

In addition to government grant or contract research proposal submissions, the raw data from government-funded projects may be subject to FOIA requests. On two occasions, in *Ciba-Geigy v. Matthews* (1977) and *Forsham v. Califano* (1978), the courts had to determine whether and under what conditions the data compiled by a private group that had received money under a federal grant-in-aid program became agency records because the federal agency had funded the project and had authority to demand those records. Both courts held that the information did not have to be released. The courts came to this decision because the projects were conceived and organized privately, and there were no substantial federal supervision and control over the actual conduct of the studies. Thus, regardless of the federal funds received by the researchers, they were not governmental agencies. Furthermore, although the researchers' grant documents established the right of access for the granting agency to the records of the grantees for audits and other purposes, the court held that the raw data sought did not qualify as agency records before the exercise of that right by the granting agency.

The Forsham case was eventually heard by the U.S. Supreme Court (*Forsham v. Harris,* 1980). That Court substantially affirmed the holding of the lower court as follows: "data generated by a privately controlled organization which has received grant funds from an agency . . . , but which . . . [have] not at any time been obtained by the agency, are not 'agency records' accessible under the FOIA" (p. 178). The Court noted that Congress, by excluding private grantees from the definition of "agency," had demonstrated an intent to preserve their autonomy by exempting them from FOIA disclosure obligations. The Court held that neither the federal funding nor the federal supervision was sufficient to transform the researchers' private documents into agency records.

These considerations do not conclude the inquiry. Although it is clear that neither federal funding nor federal supervision is sufficient to transform private documents into agency records, it is equally clear that data generated by private grantees may become "agency records" at some point. Efforts to delineate that point accurately must necessarily look at congressional intent. The act's definition of "agency" and congressional policy toward grantee records indicate that Congress did not intend grant supervision short of government control to render the documents "agency records." Moreover, congressional policy also reveals a determination to keep federal grantees free from the direct obligatory requirements of the FOIA. Thus, in ascertaining the intended expanse of the term "agency records" the act must be construed in light of the dual congressional intentions of increasing public access to government records and retaining grantee autonomy (*Forsham v. Harris,* 1980, p. 182).

In an attempt to clarify the scope of the term "agency record" in a way that coincides with congressional intent, the Supreme Court has advanced a "control" test. Control seems to mean that an agency must "obtain or create" a record and reduce it to actual physical possession before it qualifies as an "agency record." Thus, if a situation arises in which the government is found by the courts to have been involved "substantially" in the "core" of a program, the courts may well decide that the raw data are agency records and must be disclosed, despite their being privately possessed by the researcher.

Prudent researchers who seek to prevent intrusion into their research are therefore well advised to minimize both governmental involvement in the day-to-day management of the project and opportunities for the government to have "substantial" contact with the actual research documents. Consequently, researchers should consider submitting summaries of raw data rather than the actual records wherever possible and should agree to *on-site* audits of programs so that records are not removed from their possession. This may be difficult in view of the recently adopted practice of some governmental agencies that requires the filing of data with the agency as a condition of receipt of funds. If the government requests an independent analysis of data, the best protection is to contract for such services with an independent, outside party rather than submit the data to the agency for its perusal (Morris et al., 1981).

There are times, of course, when the creation of an agency record cannot be avoided. When those instances arise, it is worth remembering that the FOIA allows anyone, including the press, access to agency records. Such access to reports, combined with the fact that results so reported frequently have not yet undergone peer review or other outside scrutiny, militates against the inclusion in communications to the granting agency of preliminary data analyses or unsupported speculation about the conclusions that might be drawn when data analyses are complete. Researchers' interest in impressing funding agencies with the potential significance and implications of their research, thus, should be balanced against the dangers that are inherent in the release of tentative information to the general public (Morris et al., 1981).

Exempted Research under the FOIA

If the FOIA does apply to an AIDS research project, in that some or all of the research information qualifies as an "agency record," information must be disclosed when properly requested, unless it is exempt from such disclosure pursuant to one of the nine exceptions provided for by the act. Of the nine exemptions provided for by the act, four seem applicable to AIDS research particularly (§ 552a[b]).

The first relevant exemption applies to matters that are exempted by statute from disclosure (exemption 2); that is, if existing state or federal law already provides for the exemption of certain kinds of research, the FOIA does not act to override the exemption. The FOIA does require, however, that the exempting statute either mandates that the information be withheld in a manner that leaves authorities with no discretion or that the statute provides for particular criteria by which the decision to withhold is decided (i.e., what types of matters may be withheld or under what circumstances matters may be withheld).

Financial or commercial information and trade secrets that have been obtained from a person (as opposed to, for example, corporate reports) are also shielded from disclosure pursuant to FOIA. Although collection of this type of information during the course of AIDS research seems unlikely at first, social scientific researchers, in fact, routinely collect financial information from research participants (e.g., socioeconomic status).

The FOIA also exempts from its disclosure provisions intraagency or interagency memoranda and similar communications, insofar as those communications are otherwise unavailable by law (exemption 3). Finally, the statute exempts personnel, medical, and similar records to the extent that disclosure of such information would involve an unwarranted invasion of privacy (exemption 4). Note, however, that these records are not protected absolutely. The information contained therein is accessible once identifying information is eliminated.

Any of the statutes discussed in Chapter 5 as affording protection to AIDS research, with the exception of the Privacy Act, would bar disclosure under the first FOIA exception presented above. For a case applying exemption 2 as a bar to an FOIA request, see *Sims v. Central Intelligence Agency* (1980).

It is unlikely that AIDS researchers will be able to resist disclosure pursuant to the provisions relating to commercial enterprises. The court in *Washington Research Project v. Department of Health, Education, and Welfare* (1974) ruled that grant proposals submitted to NIMH do not fall within the exemption. The court was not convinced that a noncommercial scientist should be viewed as engaging in a "trade or business" and, thus, rejected the claimed exemption. The *Washington Research* court did not end its inquiry with that exemption, however. It also examined exemption 3 (interagency or intraagency memoranda [that would be subject to disclosure only in litigation] may be withheld from the public) and found it applicable to site visit reports and summary statements for application evaluations.

Of most relevance to AIDS researchers, particularly with regard to maintenance of research participants' confidentiality, is the exemption allowing for nondisclosure to protect personal privacy. In *Sims v. Central Intelligence Agency* (1980), the Central Intelligence Agency (CIA) appealed a judgment of the U.S. District Court for the District of Columbia, ordering the CIA to disclose, pursuant to the Freedom of Information Act, the names of persons and institutions who conducted scientific and behavioral research under contracts with or funded by the CIA. The court held that the exemption (i.e., "personnel and medical files and similar files the disclosure of which would constitute a clearly unwarranted invasion of personal privacy") did not bar disclosure. Although the court did not find the exemption applicable to the case at bar, the ruling is nevertheless important because of the court's discussion of the appropriate standards for evaluating the exemption's application. To appreciate the holding fully, it is necessary to know the unusual circumstances that led to the litigation.

Briefly, the CIA contracted with or funded many research institutions and individual researchers for behavioral and other scientific research involving chemical, biological, and radiological materials that could be used in clandestine operations to control human behavior. The CIA's research program included 149 subprojects undertaken on a contract basis. At least eighty institutions and 185 individual researchers participated, although many of them apparently had no knowledge whatever of their involvement with the agency! At least some of the subprojects tested chemical and biological substances by administering them to human participants. Some of the subjects volunteered for their experimental role. Others were unwitting participants who may never have known what happened to them. At least two persons died as a result of these experiments. The extent of possible damage to the health of others remains unknown because CIA records failed to disclose the identities of all participants.

Although these research operations were conducted between 1953 and 1966, new information, including the names of persons and institutions who had contracted to undertake the research, was discovered in 1977. Following congressional hearings concerning the documents, an attorney and a physician employed by the Nader group, Public Citizen, filed an FOIA request for the listed names.

Balancing Competing Interests. In evaluating the applicability of the exemption to this case, the court noted that the exemption applies only to individuals; for an agency to justify nondisclosure under this provision, the government must carry each of three burdens. The burden, incidentally, is *always* on the agency to support any claim of a right to withhold information, because the purpose of the act is to compel disclosure. First, the agency must establish that the requested file is in fact classified appropriately as "personnel," "medical," or "similar." Second, it must demonstrate that release of the information would violate substantial privacy interests of the person or persons involved. Finally, but only if the first two burdens are met, the statute prescribes a balancing test from which the interests of the agency must also prevail. To resist disclosure, the agency must show that the substantial interest in personal privacy is not outweighed by the public interest in disclosure (e.g., *Department of Air Force v. Rose*, 1976; *Getman v. NLRB*, 1971). Ultimately, the *Sims* court found that the documents were not personnel, medical, or "similar" files, and that no substantial privacy interests were involved. Although the court did not engage in the balancing test because the first two burdens had not been met, it noted that there were strong countervailing interests to consider.

The first determination is usually neither difficult nor confusing, except for the ambiguity associated with the undefined term "similar." This ambiguity leaves some room for argument. In many types of AIDS research it could be argued that information that identifies individual participants is sufficiently analogous to medical files as to warrant "similar" treatment. The second determination is a threshold issue; that is, there must be a finding of a substantial privacy interest before that interest is subjected to the balancing test of the third requirement.

This exemption was intended by Congress to protect individuals from public disclosure of "intimate details of their lives, whether the disclosure be of personnel files, medical files, or other similar files" (*Board of Trade of City of Chicago v. Commodity Futures Trading Commission*, 1980, quoting *Rural Housing Alliance v. U.S. Department of Agriculture*, 1974). The ruling in *Rural Housing* held that the exemption "is phrased broadly to protect individuals from a wide range of embarrassing disclosures" (p. 77). This range is generally limited to matters of an intimate personal nature. For example, information regarding "marital status, legitimacy of children, identity of fathers of children, medical condition, welfare payments, alcoholic consumption, family fights, reputation, and so on" falls within the ambit of exemption 4 (*Rural Housing Alliance v. U.S.*, 1974, p. 77).

AIDS research typically involves the kind of intimate personal information that, under the court's reasoning, constitutes a substantial interest in personal privacy (e.g., medical condition, marital status, drug use [akin to alcohol consumption], and reputation). In *Sims*, the court noted that, while material involving intimate *personal* information qualifies for the exemption, information connected with professional relationships has failed consistently to qualify (e.g., *Board of Trade of City of Chicago v. Commodity Futures Trading Commission*, 1980).

As noted above, once the threshold question of whether there is a substantial privacy interest has been answered in the affirmative, the court must balance that interest against the public interest in disclosure. It has been noted that the statutory language "instructs the court to tilt the balance in favor of disclosure" (*Getman v. NLRB*, 1971, p. 674). Hence, courts adjudicating such claims must give considerable deference to the assertions of public benefit from disclosure. For example, the parties seeking disclosure in *Sims* asserted that the public interest in the identification of victims of drug testing and the acquisition of knowledge relating to specific experimental projects outweighed any privacy interests.

Limiting Compelled Disclosures. Because the Act mandates fullest possible disclosure, even an agency that is "protected" from disclosure by one of the FOIA's exemptions is generally permitted to delete only those portions that would allow direct identification of individuals, such as names and addresses.[1] It is worth noting that, even if AIDS researchers are successful in their efforts to withhold identifying information, the disclosure of even nonidentifying raw data or summary statistics can lead to a variety of disastrous consequences.

A primary problem with the disclosure of nonidentifying raw data or summary statistics is the possibility of deductive disclosure. A deductive disclosure occurs where the identity of an experimental subject is deduced from the demographic characteristics or other information that has been included in the disclosure (see Boruch & Cecil, 1979). Deductive disclosures were a source of particular concern for early AIDS researchers dealing with very small numbers of research participants. Although the number of people with AIDS, ARC, and HIV infection continues to grow at an alarming rate, this type of disclosure is still a very real threat. For example, information from a study based on a small sample from a group home for runaway youth or drug abusers may be sufficiently specific to identify the particular home and, thus, the participants. In addition, al-

---

1. "Any reasonably segregable portion of a record shall be provided to any person requesting such record after deletion of the portions which are exempt" (§ 552a[b][2]).

though a distinction may be made between an exact deductive disclosure (i.e., a determination that a particular identified individual has some particular characteristic) and a probabilistic deductive disclosure (i.e., a determination that there is a high probability that an identified individual has a particular characteristic), either type of disclosure would likely make research participants extremely uncomfortable. This is especially so with subjects who are participating in research involving sensitive aspects of their lives, as is frequently the case with AIDS research.

Both types of deductive disclosure are more probable when the research at issue includes descriptive case studies (e.g., Colvard, 1967). Deductive disclosures from statistical tables, although somewhat less likely, nevertheless may occur (e.g., Eckler, 1972; Flaherty, 1978; Schlorer, 1975; Subcommittee on Disclosure-Avoidance Techniques, 1978). The work of the Subcommittee on Disclosure-Avoidance Techniques (1978) provided examples of how and under what circumstances disclosures can be deduced from single tables or from combinations of entries in several tables.

A second problem that may result from the disclosure of raw data or summary statistics concerns the FOIA's requirement affording anyone access to data. Persons who are not sufficiently sophisticated in statistical methods may incorrectly analyze or improperly interpret the data. This problem is compounded if the request is made by the media, and incorrect information or conclusions are published. Carter (1978; cited in Morris et al., 1981) provided an interesting example of such a problem in a report of the difficulties that were created when research information was disclosed under the Open Records Act of Texas, the state's version of the federal FOIA. Researchers working for the Dallas school system administered a personnel classification test to all teachers in the system as part of a preliminary effort to develop screening criteria for hiring teachers. A local newspaper discovered that the test had been given and asked for the data. The researchers refused, but the newspaper demanded the data under the state's Open Records Act. The state's attorney general ordered the researchers to release the data. The newspaper then grossly misinterpreted the meaning of the scores on the test and, to the amazement of the researchers and teachers, published articles on the front page of the paper announcing that half of the teachers in Dallas had flunked an IQ test!

A third problem associated with the disclosure of nonidentifying information is that such disclosure may hinder the completion of ongoing research. This problem occurs when information is disclosed and the results of preliminary analyses or the fact of disclosure itself is publicized before the completion of data collection or follow-up. When potential respondents discover that such disclosures have previously been made, they may be skeptical of assurances of confidentiality on the part of researchers. Moreover, an awareness of previous findings may poison the subject pool; an awareness of how previous subjects have responded to social science measuring devices has long been known to influence future responses (e.g., Kidder & Brickman, 1971).

Who May Resist or Limit Disclosures?

Finally, AIDS researchers subject to FOIA requests must be concerned with what has been termed "Reverse FOIA." This term refers to the question of whether the FOIA gives the researcher the right to compel the unwilling funding agency to keep information confidential when an FOIA exemption is clearly applicable. In *Chrysler Corp. v. Brown* (1979), the Supreme Court held that the FOIA was solely a disclosure statute and did not confer any substantive right to prevent disclosure by the agency. The Court held that the exemptions were designed by Congress to provide agencies with a measure of discretionary freedom when deciding what information to reveal. The Court, in light of the statute's primary purpose of facilitating disclosure, was unwilling to hold that it erected barriers to the release of information. Because the FOIA applies directly to governmental agencies, it followed that the submitter's interest in confidentiality was protected only insofar as that interest coincided with the interests of the funding agency. The implication for researchers is that even if their data fall under one of the FOIA exemptions, the agency, at its discretion, can disclose information—notwithstanding any objections by the researcher. Because the burden of demonstrating sufficient reason for nondisclosure is on the agency, disclosure may occur because the agency simply failed to contest it. Thus, researchers must be aware and should carefully choose their funding agencies. Researchers should attend particularly to the agency's policy vis-à-vis the disclosure of information exempted under the FOIA and the likelihood that the agency will zealously resist disclosure. The researcher, of course, should be prepared and willing to become fully involved in the agency's efforts to resist disclosure.

The only sure remedy for these problems is for researchers to lobby for either a tenth exemption under the FOIA or a special bill to protect both research proposals and raw data from disclosure. In the interim, researchers should negotiate and specify their rights to the data they collect in grant agreements. Researchers should also limit opportunities for government involvement in the project or physical control of the records to prevent the creation of an agency record. To this end, researchers should provide the government with summaries of raw data, rather than the original materials, and contract, wherever possible, with independent parties for any necessary audits or evaluations. Also, researchers should attend to the content of the summaries and be aware of the possibility that information might be released to colleagues or the press in addition to agency personnel.

State Reporting Laws: Abuse and Neglect

In addition to being subject to the duty to protect others against HIV infection, AIDS researchers may find themselves in the position of being required to report any suspected child abuse or neglect on the part of their participants or their participants' parents. In addition, research records may be subpoenaed to support an allegation of abuse or neglect against a participant or participant's parents.

All states now have child abuse reporting laws. Although statutes vary in their definition of the class of persons who must report child abuse, they usually, at a minimum, require reporting by health care professionals, teachers, and social workers. If, as suggested by the Juvenile Justice Standards Project (1977), any physician, nurse, medical examiner, or other medical or mental health professional is required to report abuse, medical and psychological researchers certainly are included in abuse-reporting state legislation. In addition, many states require "any person" who suspects abuse to report it (DeKraai & Sales, 1984).

State statutes also vary in the scope of their definitions of abuse and neglect. In part, this variation is the result of substantial differences in the degree to which the findings of abuse are based on value judgments as to what behavior constitutes abuse. Variations in the nature of the proof required to support an allegation also explain disparities in definitions. The Juvenile Justice Standards Project's *Standards Relating to Abuse and Neglect* (1977) defined abuse as occurring when "a child has suffered, or there is substantial risk that a child will imminently suffer, a physical harm, inflicted nonaccidentally upon him/her by his/her parents, which causes, or creates a substantial risk of causing disfigurement, impairment of bodily functioning, or other serious physical injury."

Most state statutes are less strict than these standards. Most problematic are those statutes that expressly call for a value judgment as to the limits of acceptable physical punishment, independent of its actual or probable harm. Some states include "excessive corporal punishment" in the definition of abuse or neglect (see New York Family Court Act § 1012[f][i][B], 1983 for an example of the latter).

Section 2.1(B) of the Juvenile Justice Standards Project (1977) defines neglect as having occurred when "a child has suffered, or . . . there is a substantial risk that the child will imminently suffer, physical harm causing disfigurement, impairment of bodily functioning, or other serious physical injury as a result of conditions created by his/her parents or by the failure of the parents to adequately supervise or protect him/her" (cited in Melton, Petrila, Poythress & Slobogin, 1987, p. 312). State neglect statutes frequently require only that the state show that the parents have failed to provide "proper supervision" (e.g., Bulkley, 1981). Some states even invoke jurisdiction if there is sufficient "immorality" to make the home unfit (e.g., Bulkley, 1981).

Because sexual abuse of children is criminalized in all states, the Juvenile Justice Standards do not proffer a definition. The drafters instead chose to rely on the various state penal code definitions. Unfortunately, most of the states that include child sexual abuse in their civil child abuse statutes do not define the term further, thus creating ambiguity regarding when sexual abuse constitutes civil child abuse.

The Juvenile Justice Standards Project (1977) defines emotional abuse as being present when "a child is suffering serious emotional damage [not necessarily as a result of parental actions], evidenced by severe anxiety, depression, or withdrawal, or untoward aggressive behavior toward self or others, and the child's parents are not willing to provide treatment for him/her" (Melton et al., 1987, p. 313). States drafting legislation regarding emotional abuse or neglect typically utilize broad definitions of "mental injury" that offer little guidance. Wyoming, for example, permits state intervention when parental action results in "an injury to the psychological capacity or emotional stability of a child as evidenced by an observable or substantial impairment in his ability to function within a normal range of performance and behavior with due regard to his culture" (Wyoming Statutes Annotated, 1977).

The Juvenile Justice Standards and general remarks concerning differing standards in state statutes are presented to emphasize the point that AIDS researchers must make themselves aware of their state abuse and neglect statute provisions, including definitions. First, they must know whether "all persons" need to report suspected child abuse and neglect. If not, then researchers must determine whether they fit into any other targeted groups who must report (e.g., health care workers). Second, social science definitions of child maltreatment tend to be substantially broader than those in law (e.g., Cruise, Jacobs & Lyons, 1994; Melton et al., 1987); thus, operational definitions used in research or definitions that are widely utilized within the profession may not agree with legal requirements. The broad and inconsistent definitions used by social scientists are especially problematic in this context because their application may result in, not only more reporting than the law requires, but more reporting than the law permits.

The likelihood that abuse or neglect will be uncovered in the context of AIDS research is particularly high for pediatric AIDS researchers dealing with the population of IV drug-using parents and their children (e.g., during home visits for research interviews or in interviews that include questions about family matters and self-care). Their drug addiction may impair their ability to provide adequate parenting. Moreover, any research population of parents with AIDS may be susceptible to child neglect because of the stresses and other factors associated with their illness (e.g., dementia). Furthermore, as is the case with any subset of the population, sexual abuse may be discovered among some research participants and/or their families. Obviously, if such abuse or neglect situations arise and researchers are required to report them, their participant population may be reduced. Participants or participants' parents may choose to withdraw from the study after they are reported by the researchers. Although such reporting is likely to help the infant or child participant, the adult participant and/or the parents of participants will likely not believe that the reporting has been particularly helpful to them (Gray, 1989).

Thus, although abuse and neglect reporting obligations for researchers (who otherwise have no duty to report) have not been ruled on by the courts, AIDS researchers should be aware of their many conflicting responsibilities in such a situation. AIDS researchers are required to protect their participants from harm arising out of research. Those who conduct pediatric or family research are faced with a particularly acute dilemma: protecting their adult participants may produce ultimate harm to children, while protecting children may produce ultimate harm to adult participants. Researchers should address these issues early and seek some resolution before the vagaries of particular cases arise. Researchers also need to be aware that the failure to file abuse or neglect reports may create liability (see Juvenile Justice Standards, 1977). Although there is no simple solution to these problems, one recommendation is for researchers to include information regarding reporting obligations as part of the process of acquiring informed consent (e.g., Gray, 1989; Chapter 2).

In addition to confidential information being released by researchers pursuant to abuse and neglect laws, AIDS researchers may be subpoenaed for information relating to an abuse or neglect proceeding under criminal statutes. Despite the seemingly adequate protective, civil statutes, compelling arguments in favor of disclosure under such circumstances support the position that disclosure should be made.

In *Minnesota v. Andring* (1984), a criminal trial concerning sexual abuse of two minor girls, the state sought disclosure of the defendant's records from a hospital's federally funded alcohol abuse crisis unit. The defendant had entered the crisis unit voluntarily for treatment, and, during the course of therapy, related his sexual contacts with the girls. The defendant argued that such disclosures were prohibited by the federal Comprehensive Alcohol Abuse and Alcoholism Prevention, Treatment, and Rehabilitation Act Amendments of 1974, and regulations promulgated thereunder, which provide for confidentiality of the records of patient identity, diagnosis, prognosis, or treatment in such treatment centers. The regulations purport to preempt any state law that may authorize or compel disclosure prohibited by the act and regulations.

The court held that the confidentiality of patient records provision of the federal alcohol treatment act does not preclude the use of patient records in child abuse proceedings to the extent required by the state child abuse statute (i.e., the identity of the child, the identity of the parent, guardian, or other person responsible for the child's care, the nature and extent of the child's injuries, and the name and address of the reporter). The court reasoned that the central purpose of the child abuse reporting statute is the protection of children, not the punishment of those who mistreat them, and the narrow disclosure which the statute compelled would not destroy the benefits that accrue when those who mistreat children seek confidential therapy programs. Because AIDS research presumably results in an accrual of similar kinds of benefits (i.e., social welfare), it is possible that this same reasoning might be applied to cases involving AIDS research.

The extent of disclosure allowed, in fact, may be even greater in research involving participants with AIDS, where the goal of punishment may be as great or greater than the goal of protecting children, such as when transmission of HIV is involved in a case of sexual abuse of a minor. In *Cooper v. Florida* (1989, p. 3) the court found that a homosexual defendant who committed sexual battery on a youth should have known that he was infected with HIV—by virtue of being homosexual. "Such reckless disregard for the physical illness and emotional trauma which would likely result to the victim, confirmed by the fact that the defendant has now tested positive for AIDS, is a clear and convincing reason for [exceeding criminal sentencing guidelines]." In this case the defendant received a much longer sentence (40 years) than normally is attached to the offense.

It is easy to imagine the *Cooper* court, with a determination to punish the offender, ordering the disclosure of records (research records if necessary) that could be used to provide evidence of the abuse or HIV transmission resulting from the abuse. In fact, a similar case demonstrates this possibility. In *County of Westchester v. People* (1986) proceedings were brought to quash a subpoena duces tecum[2] whereby the state sought production of records regarding sexually transmittable disease test results of children and various members of their families, in a criminal prosecution for sex offenses allegedly perpetrated on children enrolled in a day care facility. The state espoused the position that the existence of sexually transmissible disease in these children corroborated the evidence of sexual abuse. Opposing arguments cited the Public Health Law which provided in relevant part: "All reports or information secured by a board of health or health officer under the provisions of this article shall be confidential except in so far as is necessary to carry out the purposes of this article" (45 New York Public Health Law § 2306, 1993).

The County Court denied the motion to quash and, on appeal, the Supreme Court, Appellate Division, held that the trial court had exercised its discretion properly. The court noted the unique qualities of this case involving disclosures that had already frustrated the statutory purpose of confidentiality. It expressed agreement with *Grattan v. People* (1985), which held that the individual's consent to disclosure of records would not necessarily suffice to override the statutory confidentiality, given the public interest in maintaining the integrity of the program's trustworthiness. However, in this case, not only the children and parents had agreed to disclosure (and in fact made such disclosures during testimony); testimony was also given by treating physicians. Moreover, various laboratory reports were presented to the grand jury, and copies of available medical reports were then disclosed to the defendants pursuant to a demand to produce.

---

2. "A court process, initiated by party in litigation, compelling production of certain specific documents and other items, material and relevant to facts in issue in a pending judicial proceeding, which documents and items are in custody and control of person or body served with process" (Black's Law Dictionary 1426, 6th ed., 1990).

Thus, a statute's protections may be unavailable at any particular point in certain proceedings. Once frustrated, other interests may outweigh the maintenance of confidentiality and, according to *Cooper,* those other interests may be considerably weighty. AIDS researchers should keep in mind the *Westchester* case when reading the "Voluntary Disclosure" section of this chapter. Voluntary disclosure of information may render later claims to confidentiality impotent.

Disclosures Pursuant to Federal Regulations

Research funded through or regulated by federal agencies may be subject to federal regulations limiting confidentiality. For example, the Food and Drug Administration (FDA) has the authority to inspect records associated with any research submitted to the agency for review. FDA regulations require inclusion in the consent forms of a statement revealing the possibility that FDA will inspect the records (21 C.F.R. § 50.25[a][5], 1993). Thus, FDA requires that potential research participants be informed that the "legal right" to complete privacy does not apply in the context of research involving FDA-regulated products. FDA has the statutory authority to inspect and copy clinical records to verify information submitted by a sponsor. Ordinarily, it is not necessary that a participant's name be revealed to the FDA investigator, unless a more detailed study of the case is required or there is reason to believe that the records do not represent the actual cases studied or results obtained (FDA, 1989b, p. 29).

When FDA agents copy and review identifying medical records, those records are maintained by the agency according to strict guidelines intended to safeguard the information contained therein. Agency policy allows use or dissemination of the information only under conditions that are (a) protective of individual privacy, (b) consistent with public disclosure laws, and (c) in keeping with the agency's law enforcement responsibilities (Food and Drug Administration, 1989).

Although the DHHS also "has the right to inspect the records of studies it funds, it does not impose [this same specific] informed consent requirement because of the infrequency with which the Department actually inspects [participant] records" (Food and Drug Administration, 1989a, p. 87). When risks of this type of disclosure are revealed, AIDS researchers should take care not to characterize the disclosures in terms so broad that participants cannot make an informed decision. If, for example, participants are asked whether they wish their data communicated to other researchers whenever combination of data sets may be useful, the request is probably too vague for participants to make an informed judgment.

Voluntary Disclosure

Finally, the confidentiality of research participants may be threatened by a researcher's voluntary disclosure of such information to others without the participant's consent (i.e., disclosures not compelled by any outside authority with power to compel them). The legal system contributes to this type of disclosure by imposing few, if any, sanctions against such breaches. Such disclosures may not always be without thought or without due consideration of confidentiality, but instead may be the product of an overriding need for disclosure. For example, a researcher may consider himself or herself ethically obligated to disclose a participant's HIV status to protect a third party from exposure, even though there is no corollary legal duty to protect.

In addition, "voluntary disclosures" may occur because of ignorance (e.g., complying with a disclosure request without challenge to its authority) or carelessness (e.g., reporting results in such a way as to facilitate deductive disclosures, or providing others with information without first securing assurances of confidentiality). Wood and Philipson (1987) provided an example of this latter type of disclosure. Their article discussed confidentiality and the right to privacy in the context of HIV testing and was based on the experience of attorneys serving with the AIDS Legal Referral Panel of Bay Area Lawyers for Individual Freedom in San Francisco, California.

Wood and Philipson reviewed the confidentiality protection laws in California and noted that "the combination of these laws concerning medical privacy requires that no medical information be released by anyone . . . without a detailed statutory authorization from the patient, a proper subpoena or other order, a legal search warrant, or appropriate legal authority" (p. 21). In particular, they cited the Acquired Immune Deficiency Syndrome Research Confidentiality Act (1992), which was designed to ensure that any person tested for the probable causative agent of AIDS is secure in the confidentiality of the test. This confidentiality applies to records from research institutions. No such records can be disclosed if they provide identifying characteristics of the person to whom the test results apply.

However, the article provided examples of disclosures of such confidential information despite the confidentiality provisions. In *John Citizen v. City Health Project*[3] (p. 25), the City Health Project sent out a call for volunteers within San Francisco's gay community to participate in an epidemiological study to determine the level of AIDS infection in the community. This call requested gay men to undergo voluntary HIV antibody testing, the results of which were to be confidential. John Citizen, a healthy gay man, responded to this call. He was given a paper to sign which described the confidential nature of the project and informed him that his identity could never be traced back to his blood sample or to his test results. The document further alleged that the test results could not be disclosed by City Clinic to anyone else in such a way that the information could be identified with him.

Six months after his participation in this project, John Citizen, a healthy twenty-four-year-old man, applied for health insurance. As part of his health insurance application, he signed a broad authorization to release his medical records to the insurer. His application subsequently was denied. Investigation by AIDS Panel attorneys revealed that City Project had used a local hospital to test their blood samples. This hospital had included in Mr. Citizen's records a bill for the HIV test. When the hospital sent Mr. Citizen's records to the insurer, the bill for his "confidential" HIV test was included. Thus, presumably, the insurance company had denied Mr. Citizen insurance on the basis of confidential information which, by law, should not have been disclosed.

Legislative promises of privacy remain somewhat enigmatic. Despite the civil and criminal penalties allegedly attached to violations of legislation and the best efforts of numerous agencies to enforce them, researchers, as well as health care providers, testing facilities, clinics, insurance companies, employers, parents, schools, property owners, real estate agents, and others sometimes violate the privacy rights of test subjects (e.g., Wood & Philipson, 1987). Not surprisingly, these violations produce horrific personal consequences for the people tested. To stave off these consequences, "testing must be both voluntary and anonymous, and enforcement of privacy legislation must be both immediate and sincere" (Wood & Philipson, 1987, p. 25c). Such enforcement is particularly needed in cases where disclosures occur intentionally because of a lack of professionalism (e.g.,

---

3. Wood and Philipson offered composite case information. Some information had been withheld or altered to protect the privacy of the actual parties to the disputes.

telling family members or friends their participants' names and other confidential information).

Not only is there risk that confidential information will be released *by* researchers, there is also the risk that purportedly confidential information will be released by others *to* researchers. Persons whose medical records are used for research purposes without their consent are prototypic examples. The Code of Federal Regulations (C.F.R.) provides exceptions to the informed consent requirement, e.g., 45 C.F.R. § 46.117[c] (Protection of Human Subjects, 1992 [Health and Human Services]). One such exception applies to research involving the collection or study of existing data, documents, records, pathological specimens, or diagnostic specimens. This exception applies regardless of whether the sources are publicly available, as long as the information is recorded by the investigator in such a manner as to preclude the identification of participants.

The absence of legal requirements for informed consent, however, does not vitiate the researcher's ethical obligation to protect participants from harm that might flow from the inadvertent (or deliberate) disclosure of personal information contained in such records. If possible, the researcher should contact the person whose file is to be used and obtain consent for such use, if this can be done without violating the person's privacy. If the patient cannot be contacted, the researcher should (a) not use the file at all, (b) not use any identifying information, or (c) use every reasonable method to safeguard such information. The researcher should also be prepared to accept the responsibility and consequences of any harmful disclosures. A means of avoiding many of the problems inherent in the post hoc use of such information is for physicians and others who retain medical records on persons with AIDS to inform their patients that patient records may be used for research. Ideally, physicians would incorporate this into their informed consent procedures and would obtain the consent of patients before each disclosure (Gordis & Gold, 1980).

Professional self-regulation pursuant to voluntary codes of ethics may provide protection against leaks of confidential information by researchers who have not been compelled by law to disclose the data. Although professional self-regulation is regarded by some as a case of the fox guarding the henhouse, the consequences of disciplinary action by a professional organization may be grave. This is especially so in light of the interplay between actions by professional ethics committees and licensing boards (Keith-Spiegel & Koocher, 1985).

Public Health Reporting Laws

Perhaps the most likely form of legally compelled disclosure of AIDS research data is pursuant to public health reporting laws. Because they can be transmitted to others, for many years infectious diseases of all kinds have been the subject of statutes, regulations, and court decisions imposing special constraints on the freedom of individuals in the interest of furthering public health goals. AIDS is now included in these laws concerning infectious diseases (Mills, Wofsy & Mills, 1986).

At the federal level, the Secretary of the Department of Health and Human Services (DHHS) has general authority to enact regulations to prevent the spread of diseases across state or national borders (see 42 U.S.C. § 264, 1988; and 42 C.F.R. §§ 71.1–71.55, 1993). The DHHS reserves its broad authority to take action in circumstances in which there has been inadequate local control to prevent the spread of communicable diseases (21 C.F.R. § 1240.30). This is consistent with the traditional federal practice of relying on the states, acting under their separate police-power authority, to initiate appropriate actions to control such communicable diseases (Matthews & Neslund, 1986).

Acting within the authority of this power, many states have required physicians and hospitals to report certain diseases to state and local health departments for surveillance purposes. The Centers for Disease Control (CDC) is the federal agency responsible for the coordination of surveillance operations. The purpose of surveillance is to monitor mortality trends, identify emerging risk groups, document the geographic spread of disease, and identify areas where preventive efforts may be most useful (see Novick, 1984). All states require reporting of AIDS, as defined by the CDC, to the public health department. A growing number of states specifically or implicitly require reporting of HIV-positive test results (Gostin, 1989).

These state reporting laws may apply in some cases to AIDS researchers. Mills et al. (1986) observed that physicians, hospitals, laboratories, and indeed, "any other person knowing of or attending a case" all are required by law to report cases of communicable diseases such as AIDS. For example, the reporting requirements of Texas state: "A person in charge of a clinical or hospital laboratory, blood bank, mobile unit or other facility in which a laboratory examination of a specimen derived from a human body yields microscopical, cultural, serological, or other evidence of a reportable disease shall report the findings, in accordance with this section and procedures adopted by the board" (Vernon's Texas Codes Ann., Health and Safety Code § 81.042[d], 1992b).

Thus, any AIDS researchers conducting laboratory examinations of specimens that render evidence of a reportable health condition must report such findings. Furthermore, section 81.042(e) states:

> The following persons shall report to the local health authority or the department a suspected case of a reportable disease and all information known concerning the person who has or is suspected of having the disease if a report is not made as required by Subsections (a)–(d): . . .
>
> (9) a health professional. (Vernon's Texas Codes Ann., Health and Safety Code § 81.042[e], 1992b)

"Health professional" means an individual whose "(A) vocation or profession is directly or indirectly related to the maintenance of the health of another individual or of an animal; and (B) duties require a specified amount of formal education and may require a special examination, certificate or license, or membership in a regional or national association" (Vernon's Texas Codes Ann., Health and Safety Code § 81.003[3], 1992b). Therefore, many AIDS researchers, in the capacity of health professionals, are required to report health conditions that have not been reported as required. Although this section's requirements are far from clear-cut, presumably "health professionals" conducting AIDS research who have information relating to a reportable health condition (i.e., AIDS, HIV seropositivity) must report such information whenever they have knowledge that the required report was not made.

Obviously, the requirement that AIDS researchers report occurrences of AIDS or HIV infection among their participants significantly conflicts with participants' and, perhaps, researchers' desires to keep the information confidential. The desires of those afflicted with disease are of paramount importance because of the highly restrictive measures that often are employed to control the spread of disease. Indeed, the legality of measures to control the spread of infectious diseases is determined under principles of constitutional law that require that the individual's interest in liberty and privacy be balanced against the public's interest in health and safety. Balancing these interests in the context of AIDS is particularly difficult because the interests on each side are so fundamental and so strongly affected by the nature of the infection. For the individual, measures to control the spread of AIDS may invade privacy, constrain sexual conduct and procreation, and restrict liberty. The public interests also are compelling; AIDS continues to spread, is fatal, and no vaccine or curative agent has been developed. Thus, "AIDS poses the most profound issues of constitutional law and public health since the Supreme Court approved compulsory immunization in 1905" (Mills et al., 1986, p. 131).

Early cases adjudicating issues that relate to containing the spread of communicable disease have shown considerable deference to the exercise of the state's police power to promote the public health. For example, the U.S. Supreme Court upheld a Massachusetts law that enabled local health authorities to levy a fine against persons refusing vaccination (*Jacobson v. Massachusetts*, 1905). Choosing between individual autonomy and the common good of the people, the Court held that the latter had the overriding interest. The justificatory power of "public health necessity" in the exercise of state police power persists today. Courts have rarely imposed any substantive barriers to measures undertaken by states. Gostin and Curran (1987) provided several references to specific examples of measures that have been upheld by various courts (1987, p. 214).

Fortunately, even constitutional public health reporting laws do not disregard confidentiality concerns entirely. Indeed, most state public health statutes contain provisions protecting confidentiality (Curran, Gostin & Clark, 1986). Specifically, about half of the states now have special statutes protecting the confidentiality of HIV-related information. There is considerable variation in the confidentiality protection offered within these states. For example, some states protect test results from subpoena, while others simply require laboratories to develop unspecified procedures for confidentiality (Curran et al., 1986).

Although states seem to be moving in the right direction by adopting health provisions that protect confidentiality, none of these protections is absolute. All statutes, regulations, and policies purporting to ensure confidentiality have exceptions. An obvious exception from earlier in the AIDS epidemic was the requirement that state health departments receiving AIDS or HIV reports notify CDC of the reports. Arguably, AIDS researchers conducting epidemiological studies under contract to CDC were obliged to disclose AIDS and HIV cases to CDC when this reporting requirement was in place. As discussed previously, once these records are made available to federal agencies, further dissemination is possible.

Early in the AIDS epidemic, on at least three occasions, the CDC released lists of names of AIDS victims to outside agencies not affiliated with the federal government (Marwick, 1983). Two of these disclosures occurred within the context of research projects. In one of these instances, names were released to the New York Blood Center for use in a follow-up study on whether AIDS had developed in persons who received the hepatitis-B vaccine (Marwick, 1983). The main controversy concerning this disclosure centered on whether the release was accidental (Budiansky, 1983). In the other instance, names were released to the Los Angeles health department in connection with a "cluster study" in which investigators had established that a number of cases of AIDS had occurred in individuals following sexual contact with other persons with AIDS. In the final instance, names were released to the New York City, Los Angeles, and San Francisco health departments to eliminate possible duplication of reporting of patients who sought care in several different cities (Marwick, 1983).

Following these incidents, several local health departments adopted the policy of refusing to provide patients' names to the CDC (Budiansky, 1983), and CDC adopted a uniform computerized means of encoding names to attempt to ensure that identifying information could not be released—deliberately or inadvertently (Collins, 1984). Furthermore, a number of states have established a specific exemption to the confidentiality of HIV test results for the purpose of facilitating the conduct of epidemiological research. Otherwise, HIV reporting laws are without purpose. Epidemiological reports, however, are to exclude the names of infected individuals (Gostin, 1989).

As the definition of AIDS has evolved, additional threats to confidentiality have arisen. CDC currently includes CD4 count as a referent in AIDS diagnosis (1993 Revised Classification System, 1993). $CD4^+$ is a count of T-lymphocytes which are a particular type of cell, the relative presence of which corresponds to the level of functioning of the human immune system. Thus, any laboratory which performs CD4 tests may discover a "new case" of AIDS. This greatly expands the numbers of persons who are in a position to identify and report cases. This expansion, in turn, increases potential threats to confidentiality.

Confidentiality problems are not limited to unauthorized disclosure by agencies authorized to have access. Many statutes have exceptions to their confidentiality provisions which provide for the notification of individuals or entities other than state or federal agencies. Although early statutes were explicit in prohibiting disclosure of an HIV test result without written consent (e.g., California and Massachusetts), state legislatures have since realized that they must make allowances if they are to fulfill their responsibilities to protect third parties from unknowing exposure to HIV and thus curtail the further spread of HIV. Thus, confidentiality statutes are important not only to the extent that they protect the privacy of persons with HIV but also to the extent that they offer guidance to health care workers caught in the legal and ethical conflict between confidentiality and the duty to protect (Dickens, 1988; Gostin & Curran, 1987).

To further both of these conflicting needs, the most recent statutes broadly protect the identities of individuals seeking an HIV test, their serostatus, their medical records, and information obtained in interviews for partner notification. They also permit disclosures thought necessary for the public health. These exceptions to the confidentiality of HIV information, however, threaten to significantly dilute the value of the statutes. Idaho, for example, authorizes the disclosure of protected information without specifying to whom disclosure may be made. Decisions regarding who has a need to know the information are left to the discretion of public health authorities. Many of those entitled to notification are not at high risk. Moreover, in many cases it is unclear precisely how the knowledge disclosed can possibly lower their risk.

Although it will have changed by the time this book goes to press, a list of the individuals who, under various state statutes, are entitled to be notified of another's seropositivity follows:

1. A spouse—this does not include regular sexual partners who are not married (California, Florida, Georgia, New York, Maine, Rhode Island, South Carolina, and Texas);

2. Sexual assault victims—victims are notified if they have been exposed (California, Colorado, Indiana, Louisiana, Michigan, and Texas); in several states this applies only if the victim requests such information;

3. Emergency workers or "first responders"—the power or duty to notify is often triggered by an exposure to body fluids capable of transmitting HIV (California, Delaware, Florida, Hawaii, Idaho, Illinois, Indiana, Louisiana, Maryland, Massachusetts, Michigan, North Dakota, Oklahoma, Rhode Island, Texas, Utah, Washington, and Wisconsin). For example, Massachusetts requires health care workers to file a report that describes the incident and lists individuals who may have been exposed. Illinois requires a warning in advance if the emergency worker could become infected. Utah has a special provision that requires notification of the emergency worker without disclosure of the HIV-positive person's name or the insertion thereof in the medical

records. The Utah statute also establishes a rebuttable presumption that an HIV-positive emergency worker sustained an occupational exposure, for the purpose of worker's compensation;

4. Health care workers (Colorado, Delaware, Florida, Georgia, Idaho, Illinois, Kentucky, Maine, Michigan, New Hampshire, Rhode Island, South Carolina, Texas, Washington, and Wisconsin)—some states limit disclosures to circumstances where (1) disclosure is necessary to protect a health care worker in an emergency; (2) the worker is threatened by immediate exposure; or (3) if needed for the diagnosis and care of a patient (Colorado, Florida, Indiana, Kentucky, Michigan, and Rhode Island);

5. Laboratory workers—states require that laboratory workers have a legitimate need to know that the body fluid is contaminated (Delaware, Florida, Idaho, Illinois, Texas, and Wisconsin);

6. Funeral directors (California, Delaware, Georgia, Idaho, Illinois, Indiana, Kentucky, Louisiana, Michigan, Mississippi, New Jersey, Rhode Island, Tennessee, and Wisconsin); and

7. Schools—if a child is seropositive the school can be notified confidentially (Hawaii and Illinois). (Gostin, 1989)

Many of these provisions seem unlikely to apply to most AIDS research, but are offered, nevertheless, because of the variability in research methodologies, population samples, and means by which data are acquired. These exceptions to requirements that confidentiality of HIV status be maintained are designed for the protection of others. This protection has been explored through two different paradigms; a public health right to disclose in order to protect and a legal duty to protect. We will explore the legal duty to protect elsewhere in this book (Chapter 4). The public health notification strategies, including contact tracing, made possible by HIV status reporting, are related closely in purpose to the legal duty to protect.

Public Health Investigation Laws

A potential threat to the confidentiality of AIDS research related to reporting laws concerns compelling disclosures to investigate the existence of communicable disease. "Sec. 81.061(c)—The department may investigate the existence of communicable diseases in the state. . . . A person shall provide records and other information to the department on request according to the department's written instructions" (Vernon's Texas Codes Ann., 1992).

The Association of State and Territorial Health Officials, the National Association of County Health Officials, and the U.S. Conference of Local Health Officers endorsed the enactment of statutes to eliminate this type of compelled breach of confidentiality ("Partner Notification," 1988). They recommended a statute that would prohibit the release of name-linked information and public health records of patients and named partners, even if the information is requested pursuant to subpoena or court order. Until such protections are available, they advised public health agencies not to release HIV-related information upon subpoena but rather to respond with appropriate motions to issue a protective order or to quash the subpoena. Further, they stated that public health officials should advocate that court orders for disclosure of name-linked, HIV-related information should not be issued except when compelling reasons for disclosure are demonstrated. Finally, they noted that court proceedings concerning the disclosure of HIV-related information should be held in private, and records of the proceedings should not be open for public inspection and should be sealed following the proceedings. The proposed proceedings would be similar to those utilized with alleged law violations by juveniles, a group the courts have typically viewed as particularly vulnerable to stigma and other consequences (e.g., Melton et al., 1987, p. 292 [§ 11.02]).

Many of the aforementioned issues are resolved effectively in the model public health confidentiality statute by Gostin et al. (1987) which contains the following elements: (a) a specific requirement that informed consent be given before the release of any information or records relating to known or suspected cases of infection; (b) an exemption protecting the information from subpoena; and (c) a testimonial privilege protecting state and local health officials, private health care professionals, and other holders of information (pp. 46–47). Because they are holders of information, AIDS researchers might be included under this protective umbrella. The model public health confidentiality statute is discussed in greater detail at the end of this chapter.

Partner notification is a disease prevention tool used by public health authorities. It differs from the duty to protect, however, in that partner notification serves not only the purpose of primary prevention, but secondary prevention as well. Partner notification serves not only to warn potential contacts of possible future infection but also to alert persons already exposed to HIV that they may be infected. CDC has recommended that all sexual and needle-sharing partners of HIV-infected persons be (a) notified of their potential exposure, (b) warned of the danger of exposure, (c) encouraged to be tested, and (d) educated about prevention measures and treatment options. Specifically, CDC suggests that HIV-infected persons be instructed on how to notify partners and refer them for counseling and testing. If persons with HIV infection cannot contact partners themselves, however, physicians and health department personnel should use confidential procedures to assure notification (Centers for Disease Control, 1988).

For years CDC has used the form of partner notification known as contact tracing to control the spread of sexually transmitted diseases. Contact tracing is a program in which public health officials use their register of infected individuals to investigate the latter's contacts to prevent the spread of the infection. Successful programs for contact tracing require the cooperation of the person who is initially reported as HIV-positive. This person, known as the index case, is then asked to disclose the names and addresses of his or her sexual and drug-sharing partners. The state then investigates the location of contacts and interviews them. The information involved may reveal the commission of a criminal offense, because sodomy is a crime in half the states, and the use of dangerous drugs is proscribed throughout the United States. The index case, therefore, is potentially being asked to incriminate close associates. Current laws for contact tracing do not give specific authority to compel infected persons to provide personal information. There is, for example, no power to cite the patient for contempt (Gostin & Curran, 1987).

Despite the need for the cooperation of HIV-positive persons in revealing names and other information pertaining to persons they may have infected with HIV, contact tracing represents a deep invasion of privacy which is justified only by a clear public health benefit. Gostin and Curran (1987) argued that contact tracing is only justified in a limited context, because contact tracing within large infected risk groups would not produce sufficient public health benefits to justify the intrusion. They have cited several reasons for this belief. First, concern for the maintenance of confidentiality to protect close associates might seriously undermine efforts to enlist the cooperation of members of high-risk groups. Attendance at sexually transmitted disease and drug dependency treatment clinics or counseling sessions may be hindered if clinics implement aggressive programs in contact investigation. In addition, AIDS research would be hampered if researchers were required to conduct contact tracing or, if by reporting HIV-infected persons, the state public health department attempted aggressive contact tracing on its own.

Contact tracing among high-risk groups would not be feasible in areas with a high reservoir of infection. In many major cities in the United States, such as New York or San Francisco, high-risk groups in essence have been saturated with HIV infection. Contact tracing in such circumstances is futile because it would lead the investigator to virtually every member of the high-risk group. The alternative of providing major resources for public education, testing, counseling, and treatment on a voluntary basis, targeted at the risk group as a whole, would be both more effective and economical.

A systematic program of contact tracing in areas of high infection would drain limited public health resources and be exceedingly difficult to plan and enforce. A voluntary system of testing and counseling infected individuals to inform their own contacts provides the best opportunity for impeding the spread of HIV in these groups. The case for contact tracing is strongest in cities and states with a low incidence of HIV infection or where the suspected mode of transmission is heterosexual. In such cases, the contact may be unaware that he or she has been exposed to the virus. Contact tracing would allow the contact to modify his or her behavior based on the test result as explained by a trained health counselor. For example, the partner of an IV drug user could take precautions not to bear children if she has a positive serological status (Centers for Disease Control, 1985a).

If and when contact tracing is justified, two complementary notification processes can be used to identify partners—patient referral and provider referral. With patient referral, persons infected with HIV choose to inform their own partners directly of their risk of infection. Trained health department personnel can help instruct patients how to inform sex and needle-sharing partners sensitively about their potential risk for infection. With provider referral, infected patients request assistance in notifying some or all of their partners; they voluntarily provide names, descriptions, and addresses so that notification can be carried out by trained health department staff. This process is designed to protect the anonymity of patients; their names are never revealed to sex or needle-sharing partners.

Model Statutes

Gostin (1989) recommended that all states consider implementing a model substantially similar to the New York Testing Confidentiality Act of 1988 when introducing statutory confidentiality protections for HIV testing. The model statute requires informed consent for HIV testing, pretest and posttest counseling, and heightened protection of confidentiality. Health care professionals, public health officials, and presumably AIDS researchers would have the power, but not a duty, to notify sexual or needle-sharing partners if those individuals reasonably believe that the partner is in danger of infection and would not be warned by the patient after counseling on the need to notify. This balance between the importance of confidentiality and the protection of third parties has been supported by the Association of State and Territorial Health Officers (1987), among others.

Removing the Duty to Protect

By giving "health care professionals" and, by extension, researchers the power to exercise discretion, instead of a duty, it shields them from liability for failure to warn a third party in immediate danger—a topic discussed in Chapter 4 (see also *Gammill v. United States*, 1984). AIDS researchers should also be aware of two other potential sources of liability—failure to disclose as required and failure to maintain confidentiality through disclosures. For example, in Texas:

> Sec. 81.049. Failure to Report; Criminal Penalty
> (a) A person commits an offense if the person knowingly fails to report a reportable communicable disease or health condition under this subchapter.
> (b) An offense under this section is a class B misdemeanor. (Vernon's Texas Codes Ann., Health and Safety Code, 1992b).

Although on the books, prosecutorial attention is rarely given to enforcement of public health reporting laws (Hershey, 1976), and there are no known cases of anyone being fined or imprisoned for failure to report a case of AIDS or another communicable disease.

Eliminating the Liability Dilemma

AIDS researchers should be especially concerned by a state of statutory affairs existing in some jurisdictions that imposes liability both for inappropriate disclosures and for an inappropriate failure to disclose. We have already discussed at some length issues relating to liability that is imposed for failure to comply with the duty to protect. However, it is worth remembering that liability may be imposed for breaking a confidence (e.g., *Alberts v. Devine*, 1985), even though the breach occurs in an effort to comply with the duty to protect.

Texas, for example, provides for both civil (i.e., Vernon's Texas Codes Ann., Health and Safety Code § 81.104, 1992b) and criminal liability (Vernon's Texas Codes Ann., Health and Safety Code § 81.103, 1992b) for injuries resulting from violations of confidentiality provisions. Also confronting the researcher, however, are criminal penalties for a failure to make known reportable diseases (e.g., Vernon's Texas Codes Ann., Health and Safety Code § 81.049, 1992b).

At first glance, this scheme seems to establish a "liable if you do," "liable if you don't" dilemma vis-à-vis disclosures. In fact, however, these complementary provisions do not operate to penalize *any* decision a researcher might make. Rather, they circumscribe narrowly the disclosure boundaries in such a way as to limit severely the degree of freedom available to researchers (i.e., "liable if you do *and* the statute says you shouldn't have" and "liable if you don't *and* the statute says you should have"). Obviously, great conflict is generated by these competing sources of liability. The message for researchers seems to be that they must disclose enough information to public health authorities to comply with the requirements of the law, but they are prohibited from disclosing more. This statutory scheme underscores the importance of knowing precisely how a particular jurisdiction has defined both the duty to maintain confidentiality and the duty to protect others.

The Requirement of Informed Consent

The model statute proposed by Gostin (1989), in its requirement of informed consent and a description of intended disclosures before participation, along with the removal of any "duty to disclose" HIV status would help solve this potential conflict. That is, informed consent to participation in research involving the risk of disclosure under certain, clearly specified, circumstances constitutes consent to disclose should those circumstances materialize, while the removal of the "duty to disclose" removes one horn of the dilemma. Clearly, of course, this tilts the balance in favor of maintaining confidentiality, at least with regard to borderline cases.

Conclusion

In summary, a number of threats to the confidentiality of research information exist. These include subpoenas, federal regulations applicable to agencies from whom researchers may acquire funds (e.g., FDA), and various mandatory reporting laws. Subpoenas are unlikely to create many problems for AIDS researchers. They are issued infrequently, but once issued, they are potentially devastating to confidentiality. Those researchers studying pharmacological interventions would seem to be at greatest risk because of the trend involving subpoenas in product liability cases.

Researchers who receive funds from federal agencies should familiarize themselves with the extent to which such funds are contingent on agreement that the agency retains the right to inspect data. Federal agencies rarely audit research information in ways that compromise confidentiality. Nevertheless, knowledge of agency policy can avert misunderstandings and other problems that might arise once research is underway.

Mandatory reporting laws may be the most relevant to AIDS researchers. Whether those laws are likely to affect AIDS researchers depends largely on the type of research being conducted. Obviously, researchers whose participants include children and families are more likely to be affected by child abuse reporting laws than are researchers whose work does not involve those populations. Moreover, research with individuals who are at higher risk is more likely to involve health reporting laws than is research with individuals at lower risk.

Researchers should be aware of the various threats to confidentiality and the situations most likely to lead to the realization of those threats. Thus prepared, researchers can determine the appropriate course of action to maximally establish and preserve confidentiality.

Chapter 4

THE DUTY TO PROTECT
THIRD PARTIES

Melton (1991b) has observed the utility of explaining legal concepts through the use of analogous colloquialisms. The tension underlying the duty to protect third parties is amenable to this treatment. The two interests that compete in this context are the privacy inherent in communications between researchers and research participants and the duty to take steps to protect innocent third parties from harm that may be directed toward them. As previously, this issue will be illustrated in the context of AIDS research, despite the much broader scope of the issue.

The privacy associated with communications between AIDS researchers and AIDS participants is similar to privacy concerns underlying communications that occur in the context of other intimate relationships. The issue may be translated into "This is between you and me." We typically recognize the value of this kind of communication by legally protecting the right to keep it "between you and me." The legal system, however, also addresses the converse of the right to keep information between parties, namely, the right to be informed that information will not be kept between them. The Miranda warnings applicable in certain criminal contexts, for example, are primarily a mechanism whereby communicators are informed that their communication will not be kept between the parties. Thus, our legal system recognizes the importance of keeping private communications private and, in cases where this is not possible, of alerting individuals to the fact that information may be divulged.

There are many examples of reluctance on the part of our legal system to impose legal duties where moral duties clearly exist. For example, if an individual watched a bridge wash away five minutes before a school bus loaded with children was scheduled to cross the bridge, our system would impose no duty on that person to take steps to avert the forthcoming tragedy. The person could get a lawn chair, take a seat on the side of the road, and wait for the event. Although this conduct would be legal, few would argue that it was moral. The underlying issue may be translated, "You can't sit back and do nothing." This is the kind of concern that has motivated legislators and courts to impose duties to protect third parties from harm. Although the motivation underlying the duty is certainly understandable, the duty nevertheless has been met with considerable criticism.

The American Medical Association (American Medical Association, Council on Ethical and Judicial Affairs, 1988), the American Psychological Association (Morin, 1987), and others (e.g., Gray, 1989; Melton, 1988) have expressed concern that psychologists and medical professionals have a "duty to warn" third parties about possible HIV infection from a patient, client, or research participant. Belitsky and Solomon (1987) interpreted the "duty to warn" as meaning that "a physician with knowledge of a diagnosis of AIDS who fails to disclose the information to a foreseeable victim could be found liable" (p. 203). No aspect of AIDS policy has attracted more attention than the legal and ethical propriety of intrusions into the privacy and autonomy of individuals infected with HIV to protect specific third parties or the general public (e.g., Association of State and Territorial Health Officers, 1987).

Legal Origins of the Duty

Tarasoff and Beyond

Any legal duty for AIDS researchers and others to take steps to protect third parties from HIV infection by research participants would likely be based on the *Tarasoff* decision (*Tarasoff v. Regents of University of California*, 1976). Many understood *Tarasoff* to mean three things: (a) there is a duty to protect third parties from harm, which is met by warning them of dangers posed by clients or patients; (b) that duty applies to all mental health and medical professionals; and (c) the applicable duty owing to third parties is that which was judicially imposed by the *Tarasoff* court. In fact, *Tarasoff* held none of these. First, *Tarasoff* imposed a duty to protect third persons from certain foreseeable harms (i.e., *serious* dangers of *violence*). That duty to protect may or may not be discharged by warning. Second, the ruling issued from the California Supreme Court and is not binding in other states. Many other states may have their own judicially imposed or statutory duty to protect third parties—a duty that sometimes differs from the *Tarasoff* duty. Thus, researchers must keep abreast of current statutes and case law in their jurisdictions. This diversity of approach may necessitate consultation with attorneys.

The *Tarasoff* decision dealt with the duty of therapists to protect third parties from therapists' clients in certain circumstances. Although the applicability of this decision is by no means universal, the facts of the case and reasoning of the court are worthy of consideration as illustrative of the kinds of issues that concern the courts and the manner in which they are resolved. Moreover, as mentioned previously, any duty to protect imposed on researchers would likely be based on the *Tarasoff* decision.

Tarasoff involved the killing of a young woman by her former boyfriend, who had been a patient of a University Counseling Center. Asserting negligence by the center, the woman's parents brought suit. After being heard three times at various levels of the California judicial system, including the California Supreme Court (*Tarasoff v. Regents of the University of California*, 1974 [hereafter *Tarasoff I*]), which found the defendants liable for negligence on a theory of failure to warn, the case was reheard by the California Supreme Court (*Tarasoff v. Regents of the University of California*, 1976 [hereafter *Tarasoff II*]). On rehearing, the decision in *Tarasoff I* was upheld, but the basis for the decision was modified. This final decision held that,

> when a therapist determines, or pursuant to the standards of his profession should determine, that his patient presents a serious danger of violence to another, he incurs an obligation to use reasonable care to protect the intended victim against such danger. The discharge of this duty may require the therapist to take one or more of several steps, depending upon the nature of the case. Thus it may call for him to warn the intended victim or others likely to apprise the victim of the danger, to notify the police, or take whatever other steps are reasonably necessary under the circumstances. (*Tarasoff II*, p. 340)

Several standards are set forth in this holding. Note that therapists may be held liable even if they do not determine their client to be a threat to another. It is enough that therapists applying professional standards *should have* discovered the danger (*Jablonski ex rel. Pahls v. United States*, 1983).

A more recent Vermont case addressed the standard to which the professional is held. The *Peck* court held that all mental health professionals working in an organized setting, such as a community mental health center, may be held to some hybrid, universal standard (*Peck v. Counseling Service of Addison County, Inc.,* 1985). This holding runs counter to the generally accepted legal rule that mental health professionals are held to the standard expected of their discipline. Courts following this reasoning thus might hold a person with a newly received Master of Arts degree in counseling to the same standard as a doctoral-level clinician with twenty years of experience.

Not only is it unclear whether and, if so, the extent to which a duty imposed on therapists applies to researchers but also it is uncertain whether a duty to protect third parties against threats of intended violence should be extended to apply to third parties against whom neither violence nor harm is intended. We will return to this topic later in this chapter.

Applicability to AIDS Research

In addition to the significant differences between the conduct that gives rise to harm in the case of HIV transmission and the conduct at issue when violence is intended or when, because of impairments in cognitive functioning, violence is likely (whether or not it is intended), there are also differences in the predictions of each. Not only might the motivations of the infected party change the calculation of dangerousness to another,[1] but also the variability of transmission must be taken into account. Moreover, the latency period between HIV infection and seropositivity, combined sometimes with the inaccessibility of serostatus records (particularly for nonmedical clinicians), undermines the level of certainty with which a researcher can determine that a particular research participant poses any risk of HIV infection at all. These somewhat unique contours of work with people with AIDS and HIV infection necessitate further exploration to determine the extent to which the *Tarasoff* duty applies in this context.

The duty to protect applies only if a patient or client poses a serious danger of bodily harm to another and by extension should apply to researchers only if their research participants pose a similar serious risk.

---

1. It is worth noting that Tarasoff's killer intended to kill his victim. Such a clear intention to commit violence necessarily increases the probability of harm, at least when the prospective offenders possess the means of carrying out that intent. Other cases may involve no such intention to harm but, nevertheless, pose serious risks to others. For example, an individual whose cognitive abilities are impaired may believe that throwing an individual off of a building will enable her or him to learn to fly. However, absent evidence of an intention to harm or, alternatively, because of an inability to apprehend the likelihood of harm, there seems to be no principled justification for treating the conduct that is most likely to lead to transmission of HIV (e.g., IV drug use or unprotected anal intercourse) in the same manner as the conduct that traditionally has given rise to a duty to protect third persons.

Whether the danger is "serious" is a judgment call, evaluated on the basis of professional standards. The *Tarasoff* holding is based on the policy that persons should be protected from bodily harm, if possible, in certain circumstances. In *Peck,* "violence" was broadly construed to include property damage caused by the burning of a barn (*Peck v. Counseling Service of Addison County, Inc.,* 1985). Although *Peck* clearly expanded the scope of the term "violence," that expansion does not apply necessarily in the context of AIDS research. Moreover, the *Peck* holding has not been widely accepted.

In both *Peck* and *Tarasoff,* the violence at issue involved not only harm (economic and physical, respectively) but also the intent to bring about harmful consequences (as opposed to merely the intent to engage in conduct from which harm results). The question of whether a person infected by HIV who intends to have sex or share a needle with another person is intending to act violently is still unanswered.

Assessment of the Probability of Harm

The prevention of AIDS is distinguishable from the prevention of violence (Girardi, Keese, Traver & Cooksey, 1988). First, when a client or patient has a gun, an intended victim, and a vociferously expressed intent to kill the particular individual, the foreseeability of harm is arguably substantially greater than a circumstance in which an HIV-infected participant admits to prior unprotected sexual relations and the intention to engage in such relations in the future with a particular, identified individual. The lethality of AIDS and the inappropriateness of risky sexual behavior notwithstanding, intercourse with an HIV-infected person often results in no harm to the partner because of the biological variability involved in infection by the AIDS virus (Curran et al., 1988). Variability in transmission rates, however, may be a weak argument for researchers seeking to obviate a duty to protect a third party, for as Melton (1988) observed, "if the client is known with certainty to be infected, then the prediction of danger to a third party is largely a matter of behavioral prediction" (p. 942). Behavioral predictions, however inaccurate they might be, typically have been regarded as being within the purview of mental health professionals (see, e.g., *Barefoot v. Estelle,* 1983; *Jurek v. Texas,* 1976; Melton et al., 1987, § 7.06).

Although behavioral predictions regarding future dangerousness to others are nearly always tenuous (Melton et al., 1987, § 7.10; but cf.

Monahan, 1993), there are qualitative differences between the assessments of future dangerousness to another by way of violence and dangerousness to another by way of infection by HIV. The harm from being the target of a gunshot is virtually certain. In addition, whereas victims of violence may be taken completely by surprise, which leaves them with little opportunity to protect themselves, sexual partners and needle sharers by now should be aware of the potential for HIV transmission and share at least some of the responsibility for its prevention (Melton, 1988). In fact, such awareness ideally should prompt individuals to ask the person with HIV-infection whether he or she is infected and/or use protective measures, such as a condom or syringe cleaning, before engaging in such behavior, thereby reducing the potential for transmission.

Admittedly, these descriptions of ready acceptance of responsibility for prevention, effective communication between prospective transmitters and recipients of the virus, and the willing adoption of protective strategies are somewhat idyllic. Not surprisingly, research has indicated that the actual state of affairs has been considerably less than ideal. Some individuals, particularly adolescents, may not have adequate awareness of risk of HIV infection to understand the need to take precautions (Huszti & Chitwood, 1989). Of those young people who are aware of the risks of HIV infection, an alarming number fail to modify risky sexual behavior (MacDonald et al., 1990).

Between June 1985 and December 1988, nearly 700,000 volunteer blood donors in Washington, D.C., were screened for HIV infection. Of the 284 who tested positive, 156 were studied. All of the donors who had been exposed to HIV through heterosexual activity ($n = 33$) claimed to be unaware that their behavior had placed them at risk. This finding was true even for the donors who knew that their partners had used intravenous drugs or had engaged in prostitution. Unfortunately, HIV infection usually goes unrecognized (especially among women), even in high-prevalence communities (Schoenbaum & Webber, 1993).

Communication, although desirable, is of questionable effectiveness in view of the proportion of individuals who are willing to mislead potential sexual partners about their serostatus to engage in sexual relations (Cochran & Mays, 1990). All of these findings militate against excessive reliance on individuals who are at risk to protect themselves from infection. The danger of HIV infection of third parties by research participants, despite efforts to the contrary, may remain sufficient to trigger the duty to protect.

Intended Victim Requirement

Both the *Tarasoff* and *Peck* decisions contained language alluding to danger to "another" and protection of the "intended victim" (e.g., *Tarasoff II*, p. 340). This language implies that the duty of care extends only to situations involving a specific threat to a specific individual, not to statistically probable victims (Gostin, Curran & Clark, 1987). Most post-*Tarasoff* courts that have considered the issue have further limited the definition of "reasonable foreseeability" to those instances in which there is a specific, clearly identifiable, intended victim (*Brady v. Hopper*, 1983).

Some courts do not require that there be an identifiable victim for liability to attach (*Lipari v. Sears, Roebuck & Co.*, 1980; *Currie v. United States*, 1987). In *Lipari*, the court held that liability is established by the existence of foreseeable danger to any member of a targeted class of people. Obviously, there are tremendous implications in AIDS research for this type of affected-class reasoning. An example is a researcher studying HIV transmission rates among male prostitutes who possesses the "duty to protect" and knows of a research participant with AIDS who refuses to do anything to prevent the spread of HIV to others. Because several persons constituting a targeted class (i.e., recipients of male prostitutes' services) are in danger of contracting the virus from the person with AIDS, the individual seems duty-bound to contact the authorities (e.g., health department, police, or both) to fulfill the obligation. This issue is discussed in greater detail in the section entitled "scope of the duty."

Discharging the Duty

If the duty to protect third parties applies to an AIDS researcher, that individual incurs an obligation to use "reasonable care" to "protect" the intended victim from such danger. Thus, even if *Tarasoff* does apply to risks of HIV infection, the oft-cited "duty to warn" potential "victims" of infected "clients" is probably nonexistent. Other action may suffice if a researcher reasonably believes that an HIV-infected subject is not following authoritative risk reduction modifications of otherwise risky behavior (Melton, 1988). Unfortunately, this reasoning gives researchers little practical guidance as to particular legal responsibilities regarding their duty to protect. Gostin et al. (1987) speculated that professionals will not be held liable unless they are able to control the dangerous situation by initiating procedures for criminal or civil confinement or by warning those in a position to take protective measures (*Hasenei v. United States*, 1982; *Lund-*

gren v. Fultz, 1984). Whether the particular course of action is deemed appropriate again may depend on what a reasonable professional would do in the particular situation.

Although the precise steps to be taken are unclear, Gostin and Curran (1987) suggested that they at least include a threshold obligation to advise participants of researchers' responsibility to warn close contacts about the HIV status of clients. Gostin and Curran advised physicians to notify an HIV-positive patient's sexual contacts of the patient's seropositivity only when there are *strong* grounds for believing that a specific *contact* has *not been informed* and is *in serious danger* of exposure to HIV. Fulero (1988) aptly pointed out that if researchers owe a duty to third persons, surely clients should be so informed at the outset under the doctrine of informed consent. However, this action may result in the refusal by participants to reveal sensitive information or to participate in research at all. The resulting loss of benefits from psychosocial education and/or advances in research may place the public in greater peril (Gurevitz, 1977).

Duty to Commit?

Melton (1988) voiced concern elsewhere that pressure to take action greater than the minimum steps outlined by Gostin and Curran may mount and result in an exercise of involuntary civil commitment power[2] as a de facto quarantine measure when persons infected with HIV are believed to be engaging in risky behavior. Such legal action is most likely to occur in those jurisdictions which recognize substance abuse as a threshold condition for civil commitment (e.g., Nebraska Mental Health Commitment Act of 1976, §§ 83–1009 and 83–1009.02, 1992) and in cases in which the means of transmitting HIV was through needle sharing (Hafemeister & Amirshahi, 1992). The substance abuse criterion, however, does not foreclose the possibility of commitment of persons who are HIV positive but do not meet commitment criteria for substance abuse. The state may well argue that the very act of engaging in unprotected intercourse or sharing needles by individuals who know they are infected by HIV is indicative of mental disorder (Melton, 1988).

However, Melton (1988) pointed out that both of these lines of argument are seriously flawed. In the former instance, it would be difficult

2. "The proceedings directing confinement of a mentally ill or incompetent person for treatment. Commitment proceedings may be either civil or criminal; and voluntary or involuntary. Due process protections are afforded to persons involuntarily committed. . . ." (Black's Law Dictionary 273, 6th ed., 1990).

to prove that imminent dangerousness is directly the result of substance abuse, even if such a causal nexus can be established for HIV infection. If mental illness is the threshold condition, using dangerous behavior as evidence of mental illness is tautological. Commitment statutes require both mental illness and dangerousness. Dangerousness, without more, cannot serve as the basis for commitment. A state's attempt at categorizing dangerousness as both dangerousness and a mental disorder would clearly circumvent the intention of those statutes by rendering the mental disorder requirement meaningless.

Moreover, as the American Psychological Association argued and the Fourth Circuit Court of Appeals held in a recent case (*Currie v. United States,* 1987), *Tarasoff* does not create a duty to commit; one who believes an individual to be dangerous but not committable (e.g., exhibiting aggressive behavior but not mentally ill within the meaning of the commitment statute) may take other protective action (e.g., warning potential victims). Otherwise, the *Tarasoff* doctrine could be extended effectively to include a duty of care to all persons, not just identifiable potential victims.

The Fourth Circuit also noted that a "duty to commit" would contravene public policy because of the level of restrictiveness of liberty entailed. The *Tarasoff* court struggled with balancing the competing interests of protection of citizens on the one hand and the value of maintaining the confidentiality of therapeutic relationships on the other. The court ultimately concluded that the benefits to citizens in danger were worth acquiring even if this acquisition was at some expense to the therapeutic relationship. The Fourth Circuit's reasoning in *Currie* suggests that balancing the benefits to citizens in danger against individual liberties (i.e., instead of the therapeutic relationship) alters the outcome; protection in this context may be facilitated at the expense of therapy, but not at the expense of individual liberties. The question of how the balance is struck when the benefits to citizens at risk are weighed against the benefits derived from AIDS research remains unanswered. The issue is an important one because the existence of such a duty might be a particularly potent deterrent with regard to participation in AIDS research involving behavioral questions.

In short, even in cases that involve predictable, risky behavior, clinical researchers should resist misuse of commitment authority to detain persons infected with HIV. If the plan is to quarantine promiscuous, infected persons or otherwise restrict their liberty, then such a decision should be made forthrightly by public health authorities. It is those authorities who are charged with the responsibility of containing the spread of contagious disease through the use of quarantine powers. Moreover, they will likely be in a better position to assess the risk of contagion and to appreciate the liberty interests infringed by the various levels of restriction that are available.

Thus, if the "duty to protect" from risks applies to researchers, they are required to take some type of action that is consistent with a professional standard if there is a known danger to a specific person that could be averted by the researcher's action. However, there are reasons to believe that this duty does not apply to researchers at all, much less AIDS researchers. Chiefly among these is the fact that the relationship between researcher and participant is not as intimate as the relationship between therapist and client.

To determine whether *Tarasoff* applies at all to researchers, it is useful to return to the logic that the California Supreme Court used in determining whether there is a duty to protect a third party. Assuming, as the court did, that the special relationship between therapist and client (and, therefore, a duty of care by the therapist) extends to those who are affected when the therapist fails to control the client's behavior, there remains a balancing test to determine the proper policy. Among the factors to be weighed are the foreseeability of harm (identified by the court as the most important consideration) and "the extent of the burden to the defendant [therapist] and consequences to the community of imposing a duty to exercise care with resulting liability for breach" (*Tarasoff II*, p. 342).

The cost to society of breaches of confidence in AIDS-related research may be greater than the cost of violations of confidentiality in most psychotherapeutic relationships. Discussing the risk of AIDS or transmission of HIV inherently takes the researcher and the participant into legally recognized zones of privacy. Undeniably, discussions of an individual's sexual practices and drug-taking history are highly sensitive. Public knowledge about either can subject the participant to embarrassment, social stigma, and criminal penalties. Relationships among researchers and the groups most directly affected by AIDS often have been tenuous, and breaches of confidentiality would likely intensify such mistrust and deter individuals from participating in research. Furthermore, reduced participation in behavioral research designed to discover methods of curtailing the very type of harm to be prevented, in all likelihood, would result in more harm than benefit for all future potential "victims." Thus, the policy arguments contrary to the *Tarasoff* holding take on a special urgency when applied to AIDS research.

There are compelling public policy arguments against disclosure of confidential information to third parties, particularly when there is a strong need for such information to conduct research in an attempt to solve problems created by disease. For instance, several courts have held that the confidentiality of information gathered for purposes of epidemiological research should be safeguarded (*Farnsworth v. Procter & Gamble Co.*, 1985; *In re District 27 Community School Board v. Board of Education of the City of New York*, 1986). The *Farnsworth* and *District 27* opinions recognized a crucial medical interest in safeguarding confidentiality. The progress of research depends on the availability of individuals who are willing to participate in studies. Such participation often hinges on the preservation of confidentiality. This rationale applies with equal force to research on AIDS. Not surprisingly then, the same type of balancing of interests has occurred in the context of reporting HIV test results to third parties.

In *Doe v. Prime Health/Kansas City, Inc.* (1988), a Kansas trial court permanently enjoined a health clinic from informing a divorced man's former wife (or anyone else) that he tested positive for HIV. The court reasoned that there was little risk of transmission of the disease from the man to his former wife or their children. The woman had tested negative a year after her last exposure, and the man had declared that he would not have sexual relations with her in the future and that he intended to take all necessary precautions to ensure that he did not transmit the virus.

The court found that substantial and irreparable injury to the man was the likely result of release of the information, and that there is a strong public policy supporting physician-patient confidentiality in Kansas. The court referred to two measures passed in 1988 by the state legislature regarding the confidentiality of AIDS test results and found that they reflected a policy-motivated intention "to impose a duty of confidentiality not only on doctors who possess information concerning the identity of HIV patients, but on others who acquire this information as well" (p. 1027).

An assertion that this same reasoning applies to AIDS researchers would not be unreasonable. Particularly relevant in this context is the language imposing the duty of maintaining confidentiality of HIV results not only on physicians, but on "others who acquire [the] information as well." Thus, using this reasoning, the duty of researchers to disclose HIV status of a participant to a third party would not exist, at least where there is little risk of transmission.

Other reasoning as to the inapplicability of *Tarasoff* to researchers relates less to particular parties to whom duties apply and more to the character of the relationships themselves. *Tarasoff* is based on the rationale that the nature of the therapist-client relationship is sufficient to place a duty on the therapist for the benefit of other persons. Fulero (1988) noted that the key to whether a state will follow the *Tarasoff* decision appears to be the state's position with regard to the "special relationship" involved. This is sometimes demonstrated by states' adoption of sections 315 and 319 of the American Law Institute's (1965) *Restatement of Torts* (2d). Section 315 provides that there is no duty to control a person's conduct so as to prevent him or her from causing physical harm to another unless (a) there exists a special relation between the actor and that person that imposes a duty on the actor to control the person's conduct, or (b) there exists a special relation between the actor and the potential victim that gives the victim a right to protection. Section 319 provides that if one takes charge of a person and knows or should know that the person is likely to cause bodily harm to others if not controlled, then one is under a duty to exercise reasonable care to prevent that person from doing such harm (e.g., *Sterling v. Bloom*, 1986). Thus, for jurisdictions adopting the *Restatement* (American Law Institute, 1965) position, the special relationship between the parties is the essential condition of a duty to protect.

Section 319 seems inapplicable to researchers, for they are unlikely to have taken charge of a person within the meaning of the proffered statute (see further discussion on this point below). Similarly, Section 315(b) is likely inapplicable because in the vast majority of cases AIDS researchers will have no relationship whatever with the "potential victim." It is worth remembering, however, that the therapist in *Tarasoff* had neither "taken charge" of the client nor formed a relationship with the potential victim. Unfortunately, Section 315(a) does little more than beg the question. In attempting to identify precisely what kind of relationship gives rise to a duty to protect, Section 315(a) does little by informing us essentially that a duty to protect attaches where there is a relationship that gives rise to such a duty.

The Special Duty with Infectious Disease

Although there have been no cases which have defined any such duty with regard to AIDS researchers, this void does not mean that no such duty exists. There is a long line of cases in which courts have imposed a duty to protect third parties from contracting infectious disease. Not only does that case law predate *Tarasoff*, but *Tarasoff* itself was based in part on the history of judicial support for breaches of confidentiality to protect public health (*Tarasoff II*). Thus, any analysis of the extent to which a duty to protect applies to AIDS researchers must include an evaluation of the impact of the early "infectious control" cases.

In *Davis v. Rodman* (1921), physicians were held to have a duty to protect third parties who were foreseeably in danger of contracting an infectious disease because physicians have a special relationship with their patients. The court's reasoning in that case has been affirmed more recently (*Hofmann v. Blackman,* 1970). In *Davis,* the Arkansas Supreme Court observed:

> The relation of a physician to his patient and the immediate family is one of the highest trust. On account of his scientific knowledge and his peculiar relation, an attending physician is, in a certain sense, in custody of a patient afflicted with infectious or contagious disease. And he owes a duty to those who are ignorant of such disease, and who by reason of family ties, or otherwise, are liable to be brought in contact with the patient, to instruct and advise them as to the character of the disease. (p. 614)

It seems readily apparent from this reasoning that most AIDS researchers should not be held to such a duty based on these grounds. However, it is conceivable that such researchers would be found to have pertinent scientific knowledge and, if research participants were found to be in the "custody" of researchers, the latter could be found to have a "duty to advise" those likely to come into contact with the virus about the character of the disease. As was mentioned previously, it seems unlikely that the custodial requirement would be satisfied in most AIDS research contexts. One guide may be the degree of similarity of research to clinical practice (i.e., strength of analogy to *Tarasoff*). Perhaps most studies that involve knowledge of HIV status are "medical."

Even if AIDS researchers are found to have a "duty to advise," according to current interpretation this duty (as discussed previously) should not imply an immediate and absolute duty to disclose information to third parties at risk of HIV infection. Gostin et al. (1987) argued, for example, that courts should impose only a threshold obligation to advise *patients* to warn close contacts of their infection and to behave responsibly. A professional following this procedure *should* be held liable only if patients indicate their intent not to follow the advice, and the professional takes no further action. If, contrary to the view above, the duty does require direct disclosure of confidential information to all third parties foreseeably at risk, it is likely that further questioning of the patient and contact tracing would be necessary.

The conclusion that AIDS researchers' status as professionals does not create a "duty to protect" is supported by the reasoning applied in *Gammill v. United States* (1984). There, the Tenth Circuit Court of Appeals considered whether a military physician was liable for failing to promptly report a case of infectious hepatitis to public health authorities. The plaintiff contracted hepatitis after baby-sitting a child with the disease. Interpreting Colorado law, the circuit court found no liability because it concluded that no special relationship existed between the physician and the plaintiff, whom the physician did not know. The court expressly rejected the argument that a professional position by itself creates a duty of care.

Thus, whether researchers have a "duty to protect" will likely hinge, at least in part, on whether a court finds that there is a special relationship between researchers and their participants. Given the reasoning and balancing involved in the aforementioned cases, this finding may vary, depending on the type of researcher involved and the form of research conducted. For instance, full-time social psychologists-researchers conducting a survey study may not be found to have a "special" relationship with their participants. In contrast, research conducted by physicians or clinical psychologists, who also answer questions or address issues concerning AIDS etiology or high-risk behavior, may be judged to be of a nature that gives rise to a "special relationship" between the clinicians and their patients/clients.

Researchers have long argued for inclusion of the interactions between researchers and their research participants under the umbrella of "privileged communication." Such inclusion would shield the information from compelled disclosure in many jurisdictions. The argument is based on the premise that the trust placed in researchers creates a "special relationship" between researchers and their participants, much like the relationship between doctors and patients or attorneys and clients. Interestingly, these same arguments may now be used in efforts to hold researchers liable for failures to protect. This leaves researchers, who want research information to be privileged but do not want to be forced to protect others from harm, in the somewhat awkward position of arguing that the relationship is "special" for some purposes but not for others. Efforts to advance either of these protections may occur at the expense of the other.

At this time, AIDS researchers should not be overly concerned with legal repercussions for violations of a "duty to protect" from harm by research participants. Even if AIDS researchers are found to have such a duty, which, for the reasons outlined above, is unlikely, for a plaintiff to prevail in an action for breach of a *Tarasoff* duty, he or she must still satisfy several other legal criteria.

If a plaintiff is to prevail on the merits of a claim against a mental health professional or researcher for violation of a "duty to protect," she or he must prove, not only that there was a duty, but also (a) that the duty was breached, (b) that the breach of duty caused injury, and (c) that damages flowed from the injury. The standard to which the professional or researcher will be held in determining whether there was a breach is that of a reasonable professional in the community acting in similar circumstances (Fulero, 1988). Thus, even if a seropositive research participant had unsafe sexual intercourse with an individual whom the researcher had a duty to protect *and* the researcher knew such an encounter was likely but took no steps to prevent it, the researcher would not be held liable unless the plaintiff sustained injury. It is important to note that the term "injury" may include the kind of mental anguish associated with the knowledge of having been exposed to the virus and the concomitant fear of acquiring AIDS. Hence, plaintiffs could be compensated for pain and suffering associated with a failure to protect even though the virus was not transmitted to them.

Chapter 5 includes a more thorough treatment of the issues concerning liability for breaches of confidentiality. For present purposes, it is important to note that there has been a proliferation of legislation which expressly frees clinicians (and possibly researchers) from liability to research participants for breaches of confidentiality surrounding release of information to "potential victims" about an individual's HIV status (e.g., Communicable Disease Prevention and Control Act of 1987). Courts may interpret this legislative exception to liability as expressive of a legislative determination that the costs of maintaining confidentiality are too great in cases of HIV infection. Thus, even though statutes are silent as to duties to notify sexual partners of HIV status, courts may find that the legislation implicitly creates such a duty.

Absent clear statutory authority to break confidence, AIDS researchers must predict whether courts will view such breaches favorably. Researchers making such predictions should be aware that there is some, albeit minimal, potential liability for intentional infliction of emotional harm to the party "warned" in addition to the aforementioned liability to the party whose confidence has been breached. Fulero (1988) reported that assessments of liability in this context are extremely unlikely because of the operation of the doctrine of "qualified privilege."

Several elements must be proved for courts to find the existence of such a privilege. Those elements are: (a) good faith, (b) a legitimate interest or duty to be furthered by the statement, (c) limitation of the scope of the statement to the furtherance of the legitimate interests, (d) a proper occasion and, (e) communication in a proper manner and to proper parties only (Cohen, 1979; Krauskopf & Krauskopf, 1965). Although it is probably neither feasible nor desirable for most AIDS researchers to do so, the acquisition of the AIDS research participant's permission to warn the "intended victim" removes any potential for findings of breaches of confidentiality.

The plethora of legal doctrine and underlying policy arguments on both sides of the issue make it extremely difficult for the AIDS researcher to determine the appropriate legal response when the potential need for breaking confidence arises. Ultimately, if the issue is brought to court, it will be the court that decides and, retroactively, either affirms the researcher's decision or imposes liability. As if the legal considerations were not enough, researchers must also contemplate the appropriate ethical response to such situations.

Ethical Implications of "Protecting" Third Parties

Consistent with respect for the wishes of the community as expressed through legitimate government authority, psychologists have an ethical duty to "comply with the law and encourage the development of law and social policy that serve the interests of their patients and clients and the public" (American Psychological Association [APA], 1992, Principle [Prin.] F). This principle does not end the inquiry, however. General Standard [Std.] 1.02 of the Ethical Principles of Psychologists and Code of Conduct recognizes the potential incongruence between legal and ethical requirements as follows: "If psychologists' ethical responsibilities conflict with law, psychologists make known their commitment to the Ethics Code and take steps to resolve the conflict in a responsible manner" (APA, 1992, Std. 1.02). In some circumstances, competing ethical principles may be so fundamental that they arguably justify disobedience of the law. Conversely, of course, behavior that does not violate the law may still breach ethical canons.

Consequently, a determination of the legal duty to breach confidentiality by warning third parties of their risk of HIV infection does not completely settle the researcher's course of action. Several questions remain. These include: (a) whether researchers have an ethical duty to protect confidentiality despite a third party's risk of HIV infection; (b) whether researchers bear an ethical duty to violate confidentiality to ensure the safety of a specific third party in particular or the public in general; and (c) whether either of the ethical duties listed above is sufficient to justify disobedience of contrary law.

The Principles (APA, 1992) give little guidance in answering such questions. On the one hand, protection of confidentiality is identified as a "primary obligation" (APA, 1992, Std. 5.02), consistent with "respect for people's rights and dignity" (APA, 1992, Prin. D). A breach of confidence not only harms the research enterprise but also wrongs the participant, by violating his or her privacy and, consequently, his or her integrity as a person (Melton, 1983). The harm inheres in this violation of privacy irrespective of any deleterious effects on research or negative social consequences for the participant.

On the other hand, General Standard 5.05 authorizes the disclosure of confidential information "to protect the patient or client or others from harm" (APA, 1992, Std. 5.05). If legal strictures do interfere with a preeminent principle of protection of human welfare, then, as mentioned previously, the principles provide only that the researcher "take steps to resolve the conflict in a responsible manner" (APA, 1992, Std. 1.02). The Principles apparently bar neither blind obedience to legal authority nor disobedience. The clearest guidance offered by the Principles with regard to disclosures concerns not whether to disclose, but rather, the extent of the disclosure. The language of General Standard 5.05 makes it clear that disclosures are permitted only to the extent that they are necessary (e.g., "only as mandated by law," "disclosure is limited to the minimum that is necessary to achieve the purpose").

In general, psychologists should strive to protect the privacy of their clients and to promote the welfare of individuals affected by AIDS. When compelling interests of third parties necessitate overriding the interests of those affected by AIDS, intrusions on those interests should be no greater than necessary (Melton, 1988). The superordinate principle of according respect to persons is entitled to great deference, even in the face of a compelling societal interest in public safety. Excessive disclosure of confidential information also threatens the integrity of research endeavors and their corollary contributions to social welfare. This seemingly violates the very first directive in the Preamble of the Principles: "Psychologists work to develop a valid and reliable body of scientific knowledge based on research" (APA, 1992, Preamble).

In short, the question may be not whether to warn a potential victim, but rather how to protect third parties from serious harm with minimal intrusion on the privacy of research participants. The answer to that question requires considerable ethical sensitivity. Such a thoughtful approach to problems of third-party safety in AIDS research is likely to lead to courses of action that satisfy both ethical and legal requirements, at least insofar as is possible. Both the APA and the American Medical Association (AMA) have promulgated resolutions for psychologists and physicians, respectively, addressing the issue of the disclosure of HIV status to third parties. Though not always precisely to the point, these general ethical standards should generally apply to AIDS researchers.

In his testimony before Congress on behalf of the APA, Stephen Morin (1987) observed that:

> APA endorses the concept of the provider's duty to warn if a third party is endangered by high risk behaviors. . . .
> . . . The prudent public policy goal is to ensure that in any case where a recalcitrant client willfully and knowingly threatens to spread the virus, the provider should be encouraged to warn potential victims. Such a standard would relieve most providers from a perceived obligation to regularly report serostatus. This would require a more restrictive disclosure standard that would allow for such disclosure only if a provider determines that "it is necessary with respect to preventing a clear and imminent danger of transmission." Moreover, because of the special difficulties in notification of sexual partners as opposed to notification of a spouse it may be appropriate to limit the disclosure to the latter. Finally, it may be useful to restate the ethical standards of APA and other professional mental health organizations that would require the provider to work with the client to self-report serostatus. (pp. 9–10)

The American Psychiatric Association's Council on Psychiatry and Law proposed a model law to be used as a guide for state legislatures. Their proposal extended the duty to protect only to reasonably identifiable persons and only when there is an actual threat of serious bodily harm and the means to carry it out.

The American Medical Association was somewhat more expansive with its proposal to expand the duty to protect third parties from harm. On July 1, 1988 the association concluded its annual meeting by voting to impose a duty on physicians to warn AIDS patients' sexual partners of the patients' seropositive status.

"This is a landmark in the history of medical ethics," said Dr. James E. Davis, president of the AMA, shortly after the policy-making body approved a package of AIDS-related proposals. He continued: "We are saying for the first time that, because of the danger to the public health and the danger to unknowing partners who may be contaminated with this lethal disease, the physician may be required to violate patient confidentiality. The physician has a responsibility to inform the spouse or known partners. This is more than an option. This is a professional responsibility" (Wilkerson, 1988).

Thomas Stoddard, the then Executive Director of the Lambda Legal Defense and Education Fund in New York, succinctly expressed the concerns of many that once they have the ethical authority to do so, physicians, fearing liability, will overnotify, even in doubtful situations, to protect themselves. Stoddard expressed those concerns as follows: "They are imposing a legal duty on themselves. That is the danger of this resolution. I'm very surprised that the AMA would put its members in a position of compromising patient confidentiality and subject them to extraordinary legal liability. The doctors did not think this out with clarity or precision" (Wilkerson, 1988). Stoddard expressed concern that the action would make it easier for third parties to sue physicians who do not inform them that they are at risk of infection. The chairman of the AMA's AIDS Task Force, Dr. M. Roy Schwarz, noted that the epidemic was far too serious for doctors to continue to remain silent. "Every case we prevent is a life saved" (Wilkerson, 1988).

Finally, the chairman of the Presidential Commission on the Human Immunodeficiency Virus Epidemic offered a professional interpretation of the responsibilities of health care workers in a third party "warning" situation ("Excerpts from Report," 1988). They indicated that, although rigorous maintenance of confidentiality is considered critical to the success of preventing the transmission and spread of HIV infection, "adherence to the principle of confidentiality does not obviate responsibilities to protect those who may unknowingly be in immediate danger of being exposed to HIV" (p. 16). Thus, they believed that in instances where a health care provider knows that an infected patient has refused to inform a sexual partner and continues to practice behaviors that place that person at risk of contracting HIV, stringent confidentiality protection should not prevent the health care provider from warning the unsuspecting sexual partner.

However, the Commission also believed that the health care provider should not have a legal duty to warn a patient's sexual partner in these instances. The Commission contended that legally compelled notifications of sexual partners are inconsistent with a health provider's role. The primary obligation for informing a sexual partner who is at risk of contracting HIV through the patient's behavior lies with the infected person or possibly the state health department. The health care provider's obligation in these instances is to advise the infected individual about behaviors that may cause harm to others, to counsel the patient to notify third parties, and to persuade the infected individual to behave in ways that will reduce, if not eliminate, the risk. Beyond that, a health care provider who concludes that a patient cannot be persuaded to notify a sexual partner at risk should have the option, but not the obligation, to inform the sexual partner.

The ethical contours of duties to warn third parties who are at risk of HIV infection are as muddled as the legal contours. Interestingly, some consistent themes recur. Note, for example, that several authorities urge limitation of the scope of disclosures to only that information which necessarily must be disclosed to protect others. Relatedly, the qualified privilege at common law applies only if the scope of the disclosure is limited. The Ethical Principles of Psychologists and Code of Conduct (APA, 1992) similarly limit the scope of disclosures, as do the APA recommendations relating to AIDS research and practice. Finally, these policies echo the same concerns added by Thomas Stoddard (i.e., overnotification in an effort to guard against liability).

Although a comprehensive examination of the interaction of ethical and legal obligations for each type of researcher in each jurisdiction is beyond the scope of this book, some general guidelines are offered. First, researchers should familiarize themselves fully with the general ethical guidelines promulgated by their professional associations to determine precisely to whom allegiances are owed and for what purposes. A clearer understanding of considerations underlying ethical guidelines should provide guidance in the resolution of those ethical issues not specifically addressed by the guidelines.

Second, researchers should determine the status of legislative and case law in their jurisdictions in an effort to define the extent to which the law has prioritized the competing concerns at issue. Resolving ethical dilemmas in this context necessarily involves balancing interests. Because the courts judging researchers' conduct will likely not balance those interests in the same manner as the researchers, it is vital that researchers look to the law to predict the courts' reasoning. Statutory law expresses the will of the legislature; courts consider this in striking a balance. Case law, on the other hand, provides more direct evidence of how the courts are likely to resolve the issues by demonstrating how they have resolved them in the past. This, of course, may necessitate consultation with legal counsel.

Next, researchers should determine whether their professional associations have drafted specific guidelines addressing the disclosure issue. If none has been drafted, researchers should canvass the general guidelines promulgated by their professional association. This will serve the same purposes as surveying the general guidelines except that, obviously, these latter guidelines are less directly relevant to the particular issue under consideration. Armed with (a) information regarding the role of researchers vis-à-vis others generally (as gleaned from the general ethical guidelines) and (b) information regarding legal prioritization (as derived from legislative and case law), researchers will be in a position to judge more critically the specific disclosure guidelines offered by their professional associations. Researchers finding a gap in their own professional guidelines are urged to consider those proffered by related disciplines.

Finally, researchers should balance the legal obligations and their underlying policy considerations against ethical obligations and their underlying policy considerations. It is in this balancing that ethical guidelines specifically related to disclosure of HIV status may be especially helpful in that they may define the issues themselves and propose an appropriate balance.

Privilege to Disclose

Under unusual circumstances, researchers may need to exercise a "privilege to disclose" and notify partners who they know are at risk and likely will not be notified of their potential exposure by the infected person. This privilege is an extension of the privilege afforded to health care providers. "The privilege to disclose exists only when the index patient fails to uphold his or her duty to protect others. The privilege between the provider and index patient evolves into a privilege of the provider to protect an unsuspecting third party pursuant to the provider's legal and ethical responsibilities" ("Partner notification," 1988, p. 12). The privilege to disclose differs from the duty to protect in that researchers face sanctions for failure to carry out an "affirmative duty" to disclose only with the latter (i.e., duty to protect) and not the former (i.e., privilege to disclose) ("Partner notification," 1988, p. 12).

Invoking the Privilege

The privilege to disclose may be invoked when four criteria are met: (a) the researcher knows of an identifiable third party at risk; (b) the researcher believes there is a significant risk of harm to the third party; (c) the researcher believes that the third party does not suspect that he or she is at risk; and (d) the index patient (research participant) has been urged to notify the partner and has refused or is considered to be unreliable in his or her willingness to notify the partner. For example, a New York statute authorizes physicians to disclose HIV test results to the spouse, sexual partner, or needle-sharing partner of a person who tests positive, if they believe the contact is in danger of infection and will not be warned by the infected person (45 New York Public Health Law § 2782 [4][a][3] [McKinney, 1993]).

It is not clear whether AIDS researchers would be able to claim this "privilege to disclose." However, as discussed in the "duty to protect" section, there may be legal or ethical mandates for such disclosure. A key issue for AIDS researchers to bear in mind in this context is that once those researchers disclose HIV status to public health departments, pursuant to a "duty to protect," those public health departments may then make further disclosures pursuant to the department's "privilege to disclose," or in connection with partner notification activities. Indeed, those state public health departments that seek the implementation of mandatory reporting laws often do so precisely because the mandatory reports serve as the basis for other health department programs, such as partner notification or contact tracing.

Benefits of Partner Notification

In the AIDS prevention and surveillance projects supported by the Centers for Disease Control (CDC), states have been required to implement procedures for confidential notification of sex and needle-sharing partners of AIDS patients and HIV-seropositive individuals. All of these states currently counsel HIV-infected clients who are seen in public counseling and testing sites about ways to reduce the risk of transmitting HIV. These states also counsel HIV-infected clients about the need to inform sex and needle-sharing partners of their risk of infection. Forty-eight states, Puerto Rico, the Virgin Islands, and the District of Columbia offer provider referral upon request by clients. The other two states (Georgia and Nebraska) authorize notification by health department personnel when female partners may not have known that they were at risk and/or in cases of rape or sexual abuse. At last count, approximately fourteen states have partner-notification programs that encourage provider referral for all patients. Data are made available to the CDC from partner notification activities in only a handful of states.

Partner notification data from several states reveal a high seroprevalence rate, ranging from 11 to 39 percent, among persons identified as sex or needle-sharing partners, many of whom themselves are engaging in high-risk behavior. By identifying such individuals, the partner notification process can target risk reduction messages to those at greatest risk of acquiring or transmitting infection. For a specific example of contact tracing see the 1988 work by Wykoff and others.

Risks of Partner Notification

Despite the noble purpose of contact tracing, HIV-infected persons run a significant risk of discrimination if their antibody status becomes known to employers, insurers, landlords, neighbors, or others who may perceive themselves to be at personal or financial risk (Government Accounting Office, 1989). Partner notification does not apply exclusively to willing partners.

Some states provide for compelled testing of individuals for HIV infection if they are suspected of having committed certain sexual crimes. This is done in the interest of providing the victims of such crimes an opportunity to assess their risk for infection and respond accordingly. This forced testing clearly invades certain traditionally protected interests relative to the accused. Because the testing is compelled pursuant to criminal justice proceedings which are public, risks of widespread dissemination of results and concomitant discrimination are particularly high.

Fortunately, some states have provided that when such compelled testing occurs, "the state may not use the fact that a medical procedure or test was performed . . . or use the results of the procedure or test in any criminal proceeding arising out of the alleged offense," thus protecting certain due process interests (Vernon's Texas Codes Ann., Code of Criminal Procedure,

Art. 21.31, 1992a). Moreover, statutes that impose criminal and civil penalties for disclosure of test results often apply with equal force to those victims of sex crimes receiving results of tests conducted on suspects (e.g., Vernon's Texas Codes Ann., Health and Safety Code § 81.106, 1992b). Nevertheless, because of the stigma associated with HIV infection and the potential for discriminatory action, public health officials have modified partner notification procedures to balance threats to civil liberty against threats to the public health (General Accounting Office, 1989).

Minimizing Risk

The Association of State and Territorial Health Officials, the National Association of County Health Officials, and the U.S. Conference of Local Health Officers recommend that for provider referral notifications, names of infected people should not be disclosed to their partners, and no written link should ever exist between the index patient and the partner unless there are strong confidentiality protections in place ("State and local health officials," 1988). If confidentiality protections are in place, some health departments may choose to link these records so that patients can be questioned further in the event that a partner cannot be located. If confidentiality is not protected fully, written records on patients and their partners should be destroyed after partners have been notified. AIDS researchers should be aware of these recommendations if they engage in any type of notification.

Another distinction between the traditional "duty to warn" and partner notification is worth noting here. In the traditional "duty to warn" case, the warning party notifies the warned party of the identity of the person likely to cause him or her harm in the future so as to provide the warned party with an opportunity to protect him- or herself. With partner notification, there is no similar need to reveal the identity of the person who may have been responsible for any future harm. The same risk-reducing measures are applicable, regardless of the identity of the particular party who, in fact, may have been responsible for transmission.

In addition to these protections designed to enhance the confidentiality of notification procedures while minimizing threats to public health, actual and proposed state legislation has been drafted in such a way as to maximize the benefits accruing when the balance is struck. Some of this legislation applies specifically to AIDS research. For example, California has passed legislation that outlines confidentiality standards for using the antibody test in AIDS research. Those standards require acquisition of informed consent and a description of intended disclosures before participation. The statute also establishes a civil cause of action, and criminal penalties, for violations of confidentiality (Acquired Immune Deficiency Syndrome, California Health and Safety Code 199.37, 1990).

Conclusion

The *Tarasoff* duty should not be considered in isolation. It is one component of a complex system of duties imposed on various professionals to accomplish important public goals. The primary distinction between the *Tarasoff* duty and the statutory duties described in Chapter 3 is that the latter are generally somewhat clearer. Typically, statutory duties provide those individuals subject to them with some indication as to when the duties apply. This guidance may take the form of (a) statements of legislative findings (which often identify the competing interests at stake); (b) statements of legislative purpose (which often include legislative balancing of those competing interests); and (c) a description of the individuals to whom the duty applies as well as the particular circumstances giving rise to the duty (although the latter is often not as clear as one would hope). In contrast, judicially created duties give much less guidance to those individuals who must comply. It is often difficult to ascertain how far beyond the particular facts of the case the duty applies.

Although *Tarasoff* duties are somewhat ambiguous, there is some hope for researchers. While considerable variability exists with regard to the actual balancing of interests at stake in *Tarasoff*-like cases, the interests themselves remain the same. Researchers who carefully consider these interests and strive to strike an appropriate balance are less likely to overlook important issues that may factor into courts' decisions.

Chapter 5

LEGAL PROTECTION OF CONFIDENTIALITY

We have discussed at length some of the balancing of interests that occurs within particular bodies of law. In Chapter 2, for example, we described some of the considerations involved in determining whether the risks of harm rise to a level that triggers the law relating to informed consent. In Chapter 3, in the context of subpoena law, we detailed the machinations underlying decisions to issue subpoenas. Finally, in Chapter 4 we fleshed out the kind of balancing that gives definition to the duty to protect third parties from harm. While it is true that complex balancing occurs within particular bodies of law, it is also the case that decisions relating to the scope of protection of ostensibly confidential information are informed by other substantive bodies of law at a higher level.

Therefore, researchers seeking to define precisely the status of their research vis-à-vis threats to confidentiality must look not only to the balances struck within, for example, subpoena law but also must consider the extent to which other bodies of law may be determinative. This additional step is necessary because the particular outcome that appears to be the proper result, when viewed from within a particular legal context, may vary when considered from a broader legal perspective. In this chapter we describe these broader considerations.

Statutory Protection of Confidentiality

The legal system can protect confidential data in several ways.[1] Statutes can be designed to give all or certain researcher-subject interactions complete or partial immunity from subpoenas and other forms of compelled

1. This section is adapted from Gray and Melton (1985) and Melton (1990).

disclosure. Certificates of confidentiality can be issued for a particular research project so that all confidential material of that study is protected completely from forced disclosure. The court can employ a balancing test to determine whether particular data should be recognized as privileged or if it would be overly burdensome to require disclosure. Finally, granting agencies may place limitations on the voluntary disclosures of researchers.

A statute providing for absolute protection of confidential research material would provide for all such material to be protected from every possible compelled and voluntary disclosure. Such a statute, however, would probably be overinclusive and result in data availability being curtailed severely. As we have already noted, countervailing interests in the protection of public health may justify limited compelled production and release of information to appropriate authorities. Nonetheless, participants' interest in privacy and the interests of the public, the researcher, and participants in the expansion of knowledge about AIDS are likely to be frustrated in the absence of substantial protection of confidentiality of data.

The clearest protection would be afforded by a statute barring disclosure under at least some circumstances. Several current federal statutes may offer some protection for AIDS research: the Privacy Act (1988), the Public Health Service Act (1988), and the Controlled Substances Act (1988).

The Privacy Act seriously limits the FOIA by prohibiting the disclosure of certain information to the public. However, it does not offer sufficient protection to research data. The act applies to a narrow range of situations and has eleven exceptions to disclosure restrictions. The act regulates all record systems maintained by federal agencies, including research and statistical record systems. Private record systems or those maintained by state or local governments without federal assistance are, however, exempt from the act. Furthermore, even research record systems that are federally funded but not maintained directly by the funding agency are beyond protection of the act. Only if a federal agency subcontracts for a record system that it otherwise would have established and maintained is the record system regulated by the act. Records that are not individually identifiable are not regulated by the act. Moreover, the apparent coverage of individually identifiable data is deceptive because it is difficult to determine what is individually identifiable.

Materials that do not contain names, social security numbers, or other obvious identifiers still may contain information that renders individuals' identity discoverable by inference or deduction. Thus, almost the only protection the Privacy Act does offer is against public solicitations for information maintained by the federal government that obviously identifies individuals.

Despite the general legal policy that justice demands every person's evidence (see *United States v. Nixon*, 1974), Congress has enacted a law providing for an apparently absolute researcher-participant privilege when it is covered by a certificate of confidentiality issued by the Department of Health and Human Services (DHHS). In the Health Omnibus Programs Extension of 1988, Congress amended subsection 301(d) (42 U.S.C. § 242a) of the Public Health Service (PHS) Act as follows:

> The Secretary [of Health and Human Services] may authorize persons engaged in biomedical, behavioral, clinical, or other research (including research on the use and effect of alcohol and other psychoactive drugs) to protect the privacy of individuals who are the subject of such research by withholding from all persons not connected with the conduct of such research, the names, or other identifying characteristics of such individuals. Persons so authorized to protect the privacy of such individuals may not be compelled in any federal, state, or local civil, criminal, administrative, legislative, or other proceedings to identify such individuals.

The 1988 amendment expanded the scope of potential coverage of certificates of confidentiality under the PHS Act beyond mental health and substance abuse research, for which they had been available already. The amendment was passed as part of a package of provisions for AIDS research and thus was apparently intended to provide protection for participants in behavioral-epidemiological research in which participants may be asked to provide intimate details about sexual behavior, for example.

Because of the supremacy of federal law, the PHS Act preempts state evidence law. The broad coverage—even to "other" legal proceedings at whatever level of government—also appears to grant an absolute privilege to participants in research conducted under a certificate of confidentiality. On closer scrutiny, though, the coverage is not as clear as it should be to guarantee protection of privacy.

The most obvious gap is that issuance of certificates is discretionary. Researchers often do not know that such certificates are available even for research that is not federally funded. If they do not know about the possibility, they may fail to grasp the risk of compelled disclosure of data, or they simply may not wish to invest the time in applying for a certificate. Under the former provision for certificates of confidentiality for mental health research, one of us (Melton) obtained a certificate for research being conducted on children involved in criminal child abuse proceedings. Even though the certificate was issued in the summer, it was the seventh issued by the National Institute of Mental Health that year! It is unlikely that the project was only the seventh sensitive mental health-related study initiated that year.

To compound the problem somewhat, the proposed policy statement of DHHS to implement the 1988 amendment limits the applicability of certificates to "research of a sensitive nature where the protection is judged necessary to achieve the research objectives." That provision arguably contravenes the express intent of Congress to protect participants' privacy by focusing the inquiry on the probable effects of a lack of such protection on the research, not the participants. Moreover, by requiring a case-by-case determination of "sensitivity" before a certificate is issued, the policy potentially increases administrative cost and processing time significantly. Such potential difficulty decreases the probability that DHHS will be active in informing the research community about the availability of certificates and increases the likelihood that researchers will be deterred from applying by the prospect of delaying their projects.

The protection of participants should not be contingent on the investigators' knowledge and diligence. Therefore, provision of certificates should be automatic for human research funded by the Public Health Service and the Administration for Children and Families and their constituent institutes and centers. Such research is obviously legitimate and can generally be presumed to be included within zones of privacy. Current legislation gives the Secretary of Health and Human Services sufficient discretion to adopt a rule conferring certificates automatically on funded research in the manner that we are proposing. Without such action by the DHHS, Congress should amend the authorizing statute accordingly.

Because much important, sensitive human research is not federally funded, the possibility of application for certificates should still remain, even if automatic certification is provided for funded research. However, the decision whether to grant a certificate should not be based on the level of sensitivity of the study, because all participants should be able to expect protection of privacy and because the determination of sensitivity is necessarily time-consuming and value-laden. Rather, the question should simply be whether the project involves legitimate behavioral or clinical research, the only criterion embedded directly in the statute. That question remains important; otherwise, individuals wishing to hide particular information (e.g., revelations made by psychotherapy clients who have been abusive toward family members) might establish a "research project" as a ruse to protect information gathered for other purposes.

The remaining problems with the statutory authority are ones of ambiguity in the language. Because the plain language of the statute protects *identifying information,* it is arguable that *data* of a known participant are not immune from subpoena. Therefore, to use the study mentioned earlier as an example, an attorney who knew that all children in the county who were involved in abuse cases were participating in the study might attempt to subpoena the data of a particular child.

It is likely that the choice of language was a drafting error due to the assumption that the primary problem is protecting the identity of persons who have mental disorders or who are substance abusers. Faced with a subpoena for the data of a known participant, a court probably would hold that they were covered by the certificate of confidentiality because enforcement of the subpoena would frustrate the express intent of Congress to protect participants' privacy. However, without litigation to resolve the issue, the level of assurance of confidentiality that can be given to participants involved in litigation is unclear. Therefore, for the short term, researchers studying participants in potential legal jeopardy (e.g., people with AIDS who are facing civil commitment or guardianship proceedings because of, for example, AIDS-related dementia) are advised to obtain a memorandum of law from the presiding judge (if litigation is underway) or the attorney general in their jurisdiction to indicate the applicability of certificates before their scope is challenged. For the long term, Congress should adopt a technical amendment to clarify that data as well as identifying information are covered by certificates.

In addition to ambiguity about the range of information covered by confidentiality certificates, there is uncertainty about the scope of situations in which they are applicable. The question is one of definition of "proceedings" under the PHS Act. Because a report of child maltreatment, a petition for civil commitment, or a warning to a participant's intended victim is not admitted directly into evidence in a trial or a hearing, it might be argued that such breaches of confidence are not prohibited by a certificate of confidentiality. Again, the answer ultimately must come through litigation or legislation.

However, our view is that confidentiality certificates preempt *any* compelled disclosure. Not only did Congress provide an exhaustive list of "proceedings" in which disclosure of data might be compelled but it also included language that supports "withholding [identifying information] from all persons not connected with the conduct of such research." Therefore, child abuse reporting laws are preempted by the PHS Act when a certificate has been granted. By the same token, any *Tarasoff* duty would be negated. Nonetheless, risk-averse researchers are likely to interpret the certificates as not preempting reporting laws or *Tarasoff* duties because of the liability that would accrue if a court did not accept the interpretation of the PHS Act that we have suggested.

In short, the application of certificates of confidentiality is more equivocal than Congress probably intended. Stronger regulations and minor statutory amendments are needed so that the privacy of actual participants may be protected fully. Nonetheless, as our conclusion about the preemption of child abuse reporting laws indicates, certificates of confidentiality do offer substantial protection. Even with the flaws in the current statute and DHHS policy, any researcher who plans to collect potentially identifiable data should seek a certificate before initiating the project.

Judicial Protection of Confidentiality

Statutory protection of confidential information is preferable to judicial protection of confidentiality because statutes include statements of underlying policies and the legislature's prioritization of those policies. Therefore, they provide clearer protection on which to rely. However, because many jurisdictions do not have statutes protecting certain ostensibly confidential information, researchers and practitioners must necessarily look to the judiciary. When judicial protection is invoked, the court decides whether to order compliance with a subpoena or other demand for research information. The court makes such a determination following the researcher's motion to quash (i.e., nullify) the subpoena.

Moving to quash a subpoena may be required by various ethical standards. For example, such motions arguably are mandated by the following provision of the Ethical Principles of the American Psychological Association (APA):

5.02 Maintaining Confidentiality
Psychologists have a primary obligation and take reasonable precautions to respect the confidentiality rights of those with whom they work or consult, recognizing that confidentiality may be established by law, institutional rules, or professional or scientific relationships. (APA, 1992)

Absent statutory authority for holding that research data are privileged, courts may rely on constitutional grounds, the common law, or other judicial rules for disposition of the matter. These lines of legal authority vary in terms of force, scope, and substance. Consequently, each will be discussed in turn.

Constitutional Protection

If researcher-participant communications were constitutionally protected as a fundamental right, research information would nearly always be withheld regardless of its dispositive value or the context within which the information is sought. Thus, it should come as no surprise that such privilege has never been found to be an absolute constitutional right. The constitutional contours of the issue are nevertheless important, as courts often base findings of common law privilege or otherwise protect communications on the basis of constitutional arguments. Hence, constitutional arguments may prevail, albeit somewhat indirectly.

Two amendments to the Constitution are particularly likely to be applicable to researchers seeking to assert a privilege regarding researcher-participant communication. The First Amendment is often invoked to protect information which, if disclosed, would hamper the future flow of such information. Courts are reluctant to permit this "chilling" effect on the flow of ideas. The Due Process Clause of the Fourteenth Amendment is also invoked by researchers who claim to have either a liberty interest or a property right in their research. These provisions are often used individually or in tandem to ground an argument for academic freedom.

Academic freedom generally means "the right of the individual faculty member to teach, carry on research, and publish without interference from the government, the community, the university administration, or [other] faculty members" (Emerson, 1970, p. 451). The U.S. Supreme Court has never treated academic freedom as a constitutional right per se, and academic freedom is not addressed explicitly by the Constitution. Courts and commentators nevertheless have characterized academic freedom as being at least peripherally protected by the First Amendment (Matherne, 1984).

The First Amendment and Academic Freedom. The interests protected by the First Amendment are freedoms of speech and of the press.[2]

2. The First Amendment, of course, also contains the religion clauses (i.e., Free Exercise and Establishment). However, these clauses relate only tangentially to academic freedom (to

Confidential information may be protected by the First Amendment because compelled disclosures would constrain the flow of information to the public. The argument is that the resulting impoverishment of the marketplace of ideas is contrary to the Constitution.

Few cases are grounded exclusively in the First Amendment. Parties asserting an academic freedom typically invoke the First Amendment in an effort to confer constitutional status on their tautological position. If they are successful in this regard, researchers may benefit from considerable deference as the courts balance the researchers' need to comply with subpoenas (Matherne, 1984). This elevated standard of review has been applied in several cases.

In *Sweezy v. New Hampshire* (1957), U.S. Supreme Court Justice Frankfurter asserted in his concurring opinion that "[research] inquiries . . . must be left as unfettered as possible . . . except for reasons that are exigent and obviously compelling" (p. 262). In *Dow Chemical Company v. Allen* (1982), the Seventh Circuit Court of Appeals observed that a subpoena for data collected by a university scholar would be constitutionally tolerable only when a compelling need for the information could be demonstrated. The court observed that "what precedent there is at the Supreme Court level suggests that to prevail over academic freedom the interests of government must be strong and the extent of intrusion carefully limited" (p. 1275).

Because determinations of the need to disclose involve the balancing of interests, assessments must focus not only on the governmental interests but also on the researcher's interests. The researcher's interests are likely to be at their zenith when research is ongoing and the subpoena prospectively incorporates data that are still uncollected. The ongoing nature of the research is significant because the disclosure of the unpublished results of a study is especially threatening to the research enterprise (e.g., early disclosure may jeopardize funding, publication, etc.). If data that are still to be collected are included in the subpoena, the study itself may be compromised (e.g., contamination of the subject pool, need to redesign the study, etc.). It is clear that researchers asserting such a privilege are likely to prevail if either (or both) of two conditions exist: the governmental interest is not strong, or the researchers' interests are very compelling.

Perhaps the best known application of a First Amendment argument

---

the extent that they facilitate freedom of thought and belief). Consequently, we have chosen not to discuss them.

in this context was in the case of *United States v. Doe* (1st Cir. 1972). In that case, Samuel Popkin, a political scientist, sought to protect confidential communications from a criminal grand jury inquiry into the distribution of the Pentagon Papers. He sought to ground this "scholar's privilege" in the Constitution. He was forced to justify his refusal to answer questions concerning conversations with individuals to whom he had promised confidentiality. Popkin argued that a breach of these promises would threaten his scholarly research by deterring persons from disclosing private information. This, he asserted, would restrict the free flow of information protected by the first amendment.

The First Circuit Court of Appeals framed this interest as follows:

> His privilege, if it exists, exists because an important public interest in the continued flow of information to scholars about public problems would stop if scholars could be forced to disclose the sources of such information. . . . As is true of other behavioral scientists, his research technique rests heavily on inquiry of others as to their attitudes, knowledge, or experience. Often such inquiry is predicated on a relationship of confidence.

Despite the court's recognition of "an important public interest," it rejected Popkin's constitutional argument. The court observed that the rationale for the "scholar's privilege" led to the conclusion that once sources provided information, the flow of information from the scholars to the public should not be inhibited. This, said the court, did not require protection of the sources per se. Moreover, Popkin was forced to answer those questions which related to his conversations with other scholars because his arguments concerning deterrence of disclosures of private information were viewed as less compelling as the sources of information became less direct. However, he was not required to provide any confidential information acquired in the course of a researcher-participant relationship.

In re Grand Jury Subpoena Dated Jan. 4, 1984 (1984) was a similar case involving a First Amendment claim asserted for the protection of research information acquired in connection with a graduate student's dissertation entitled, "The Sociology of the American Restaurant." A fire had occurred at the restaurant under study, and a criminal grand jury issued a subpoena during the course of their arson investigation. The subpoena was resisted, and, on appeal, the court held the following: "The application of a scholar's privilege, if it exists, requires a threshold showing consisting of a detailed description of the nature and seriousness of the scholarly study, the methodology employed, the need for assurances of confidentiality to various sources, and how disclosure will seriously impinge upon that confidentiality." Because the record before the appeals court did not address those issues adequately, the case was remanded to the lower court for further proceedings.

These cases are encouraging for AIDS researchers. They demonstrate a willingness on the part of courts to protect the privacy of research participants when confidentiality of data is necessary for the generation of knowledge. Also encouraging is the fact that such interests have been protected in the context of criminal proceedings where the public interest in information is particularly high.

Some commentators have posited the existence of a researcher's privilege, a privilege extrapolated from the journalist's privilege. In *Branzburg v. Hayes* (1972) the U.S. Supreme Court failed to grant the press an absolute or qualified evidentiary privilege. What has emerged, however, from broad readings of the case is that courts should adopt a balancing approach that affords considerable protection against compelled disclosures of sources in civil law suits to those journalists who are not parties to the actions. Disclosures of confidential sources would be compelled only upon a "clear and specific" showing that the information sought is highly relevant and critical to the maintenance of the claim and that the information is not obtainable from other available sources. Litigants rarely overcome these obstacles to discovery. Thus, the sources are shielded in all but the most exceptional cases (Brown, 1983).

Brown (1983) argued that it is impossible to make a principled distinction between journalists and others engaged in the generation and dissemination of information. *Baker v. F & F Inc.* (1972) is a case that involved a college professor who had written an exposé in the *New York Times* of corrupt real estate practices, an article later published in a scholarly journal. To compel disclosure of the source for the scholarly journal article but not for the newspaper story confuses First Amendment interests with judgments about the credibility, values, and methods of certain professions. In both situations, the public's interest in the free flow of information is implicated and must be balanced against the societal interest in compelling testimony.

This reasoning is echoed in the case of *von Bulow v. von Bulow* (1987). There the court held the process of news gathering to be a protected right under the First Amendment. This right emanates from the strong public policy supporting the unfettered communication of information by the journalist to the public. Whether a person is a journalist is determined by the person's intent at the inception of the information-gathering process. A person who gathers information initially for a purpose other than public dissemination may not invoke the journalist's First Amendment news gathering privilege to prevent discovery of information in a civil litigation, even if the information ultimately is disseminated in published form. Individuals may assert the journalist's privilege successfully if they are involved in activities traditionally associated with the gathering and dissemination of news, even though they are not members of the institutionalized press.

Thus, if researchers are able to demonstrate that their intent at the time they began their "news gathering" was to disseminate the information to the public, the constitutional protection afforded journalists will likely extend to the researchers. Given the overwhelming public interest in AIDS and AIDS research, the threshold requirement that the information be intended for public dissemination should be satisfied relatively easily.

Ultimately, however, it may be of little help that researchers possess the same privilege as journalists. As Boness and Cordes (1973) made clear, the actual, narrow holding of the *Branzburg* court was that journalists are granted a constitutional privilege only where bad faith or harassment can be demonstrated, or where the information sought is irrelevant to the investigation. Boness and Cordes nevertheless agreed that researchers should be entitled to the same level of protection as journalists, however minimal that protection may be.

Clearly, the First Amendment is one source that may confer constitutional status on the researcher-subject relationship via a "scholar's privilege." Such a privilege would be an extension of the journalist's privilege. However, because the journalist's privilege itself is subject to abrogation, it is necessary to look to other parts of the Constitution for protection of researchers' confidential material.

The Fourteenth Amendment Due Process Clause and Academic Freedom. Other constitutional arguments that can be made for an academic freedom claim stem from the Due Process Clause of the Fourteenth Amendment: "No state shall . . . deprive any person of life, liberty, or property, without due process of law." Forced disclosure of data may deprive a researcher of property without due process. Before publication, the researcher may be relying on the research to attain enhanced standing in the academic community. The value of the research to the investigator would be diminished significantly if results were disclosed prematurely and scholarly publication was therefore foreclosed.

Another argument under the Fourteenth Amendment is that a researcher's interest in personal liberty is violated by forced disclosure of data. The argument rests on the assumption that a "researcher has a personal right to conduct research free from unjustifiable interruption" (Matherne, 1984). No court yet has addressed these constitutional arguments in the context of forced disclosure of research, so it is impossible to say whether such claims would prevail in AIDS research. However, if such rights were recognized for researchers, AIDS researchers would certainly be entitled to such rights, particularly given the streamlined publishing that is taking place in the context of AIDS research.

Constitutional Penumbras in the Bill of Rights. Finally, constitutional arguments for a researcher-participant privilege may be based on participants' rights, as opposed to researchers' rights. The decision handed down by the United States Supreme Court in *Griswold v. Connecticut* (1965) is the necessary starting point for any discussion of the constitutional law of confidentiality.

In *Griswold*, the Supreme Court found that the First, Third, Fourth, Fifth, and Ninth Amendments have penumbras, "formed by emanations from those guarantees that help give them life and substance" (p. 484). These amendments and their penumbras create zones of privacy. The constitutional protection of privacy, therefore, can be said not to be tied to any particular constitutional provision, but instead is to be extrapolated from the various individual rights guaranteed by the Bill of Rights and the Fourteenth Amendment.[3]

The scope of the interests embraced by the right of privacy is as difficult to identify as the precise constitutional source of their protection. The decision in *Whalen v. Roe* (1977), however, is both relevant and informative in this context. There the Court tentatively recognized a constitutional interest in confidentiality and distinguished two different kinds of privacy interests—one in independence in making important decisions and the other in avoiding disclosures of personal matters (i.e., confidentiality). Although the vast majority of cases interpret Whalen as giving this confiden-

---

3. Although a complete discussion of the genesis of the right of privacy is beyond the scope of this book, it is worth noting that some scholars and courts have grounded the right more directly in the language of the Constitution, rather than relying on the penumbral approach.

tiality interest some level of constitutional protection,[4] federal courts disagree as to the scope and even the existence of this interest. Neither *Whalen* nor *Griswold* clearly explicates either the particular types of "personal matter" protected by the Constitution or how the interests, once defined, are to be weighed against the competing interests of the state or other individuals.

The cases that recognize a constitutional interest in confidentiality limit its application to those factual situations in which the individual has a "legitimate expectation of privacy" in the particular information at issue. Derived from Fourth Amendment jurisprudence and tort law, the "legitimate" or "reasonable expectation of privacy" test consists of two requirements: (a) the individual must manifest an actual or subjective expectation that the information will not be disclosed, and (b) the individual's expectation must be one that society recognizes as "legitimate" or "reasonable" (*Katz v. United States*, 1967, Harlan, J., concurring).

Brown (1983) summarized the interests and likely outcomes of those cases involving the balancing of privacy expectations. Generally, if a person has no reasonable expectation of privacy in ostensibly private material, disclosure is ordered without an inquiry into the state's need for the information. If, on the other hand, a person has a reasonable expectation of privacy and no strong state interests exist, disclosure of the information cannot be compelled. The more difficult cases are, of course, those cases in which a person has a reasonable expectation of privacy and the state has a strong interest in the information. In those cases, disclosure usually will be compelled.

Although courts are willing to compel the disclosure of information in some cases in which individuals do have a reasonable expectation of privacy, the courts nevertheless proceed with caution in fashioning the disclosure order. Courts usually tailor disclosure orders to mitigate potential intrusiveness and require states to use the least intrusive alternative in disclosure legislation. Moreover, it is often the individuals whose privacy interests are at stake that benefit most from the disclosure.

4. See *General Motors Corp. v. Director of National Institute for Occupational Safety and Health*, 1980; *Robinson v. Magovern*, 1979; *Schachter v. Whalen*, 1978; and *United States v. Westinghouse Elec. Corp.*, 1980, for holding that discovery of general medical records implicates the constitutional right to confidentiality recognized in Whalen. See *Hawaii Psychiatric Society v. Ariyoshi*, 1979, and *Lora v. Board of Education*, 1977, for holdings that the disclosure of psychiatric records implicates the constitutional right to confidentiality recognized in Whalen.

Courts have applied this same type of privacy analysis in the varied contexts of the attorney-client privilege, the psychotherapist-patient privilege, and the doctor-patient privilege. In these and similar cases the privileges are sustained in part because the client or patient has a reasonable expectation that the communications will be kept confidential. The mere expectation of legal protection by itself will not produce such protection, however.

Courts that have found communications between parties to be privileged have based such findings on an expectation of confidentiality by the parties. Thus, the rationale for these decisions necessarily goes beyond the law itself. However, grounding the privilege in expectations may be tautological. Key in this regard is the exact meaning of "expectation." It may be the case that the expectation of privacy exists in the first place because of the privilege against disclosure. For example, if clients (or research participants) were informed that communications with their attorneys (or researchers) would not be privileged, they no longer would have the subjective expectation of privacy on which the privilege is based. As stated by the court in *In re January 1976 Grand Jury* (1976, p. 728), "the basis for the privilege is to afford the client a reasonable expectation of privacy and confidentiality with regard to disclosures made during the course of consultations with [his or her] attorney." Thus, the expectation of privacy rationale merely begs the essential question of whether such communications should be kept confidential. This analytical problem plagues privacy law (Brown, 1983).

Despite the problems with the "reasonable expectation of privacy" test, courts have used it to develop a hierarchy of types of personal information that will be given protection. Information involving a person's sex life or health—either physical or mental—qualifies for the greatest protection. Less protection is given to financial information. Little or no protection is given to routine, biographical information, such as social security numbers, names, and addresses.

There is general agreement that "public disclosure of highly sensitive or intimate information given to the researcher in confidence can damage the privacy interests of the subject" (Brown, 1983, p. 1013). This harm is particularly salient for AIDS research. For much of AIDS research, it could be shown that the highest level of protection should be afforded research data, given the sexual- and health-related nature of AIDS and the harm associated with its stigma. Furthermore, a compelling argument could be made that much of even the routine biographical information should be afforded heightened protection because of the information conveyed by virtue of the nature of the research itself.

Although it would seem that a research participant's desire to keep AIDS research information confidential would fall squarely within traditionally recognized interests in confidentiality, this privacy claim has yet to be addressed by the courts. Perhaps this is a function of the fact that it is the researcher who is in the position of contesting subpoenas. Nevertheless, decisions on the enforcement of subpoenas of research data typically have paid little attention to participants' interests. Researchers facing subpoenas should consider the utility of involving participants in efforts to resist subpoenas in order to maximize the chances that the participants' interests will be vindicated.

Courts deciding whether to compel disclosure typically consider the extent to which such disclosure will deter prospective participants. Such a deterrent effect harms the public by constraining research and its consequent advances. This analytical approach typically ignores the privacy rights of research participants. However, this approach is not universal. In at least two cases, the courts' primary focus was the protection of the privacy rights of research participants.

In *Lampshire v. Procter & Gamble* (1982), a civil action concerning toxic shock syndrome purportedly resulting from the use of tampons, Procter and Gamble subpoenaed the records of the Centers for Disease Control. These records included "information about medical history, personal hygiene, menstrual flow, sexual activity, contraceptive methods, history of pregnancies, douching habits, and tampon use" (p. 60). Although the *Lampshire* court determined that it was unnecessary to decide either whether a constitutional right to privacy existed or its relative weight, a protective order was granted against the subpoena on the basis of the privacy rights of the participants. The court made the following observations: (a) the information obtained from the research participants is quite personal and sensitive; (b) it is imminently appropriate to protect such participants from questions by strangers about such personal matters, and (c) there was an insufficient demonstration of necessity to warrant the invasion of the personal privacy of the participants.

A similar case, *Application of R. J. Reynolds Tobacco Co.* (1987), involved the motion by a medical school, researchers, and the American Cancer Society to quash a subpoena duces tecum for data compiled in the course of a study on the multiplicative effect of smoking on asbestos exposure or to issue a protective order denying disclosure of such data. The court considered the confidentiality interests of the patients who were sources of data and held that forced disclosure would be unduly burdensome and disruptive of ongoing research. Although some of the patients enjoyed a statutory privilege of confidentiality with their physicians, others had nothing to rely on other than a promise of confidentiality.

These cases would clearly support the attempts of AIDS researchers to quash subpoenas for "confidential" research information, despite their focus on other topics. Moreover, a few cases relating to AIDS have been litigated on the issue of constitutional privacy rights. In *Rasmussen v. South Florida Blood Service, Inc.* (1987), the court held that the privacy interests of volunteer blood donors, coupled with society's interest in maintaining a strong volunteer blood donation system, outweighed an AIDS victim's interest in discovering the identity of blood donors to establish negligence in a personal injury action by showing that his condition was caused by an HIV-infected blood transfusion. In balancing the competing interests the court expressed the opinion that disclosure of information relating to donors would probably implicate privacy interests protected by the federal Constitution. The court ultimately did not engage in a constitutional privacy analysis because the interests involved were protected adequately by Florida discovery rules. Furthermore, state constitutional protections independently protected the citizens' privacy, including the citizens' right to determine whether sensitive information would be disclosed to others.

In a similar case in Colorado, *Belle Bonfils Memorial Blood Center v. Denver District Court* (1988), the court held that an individual who received a contaminated blood transfusion may not discover the identity of an infected blood donor. However, the court did permit limited discovery, void of personal identifiers, to determine whether the blood bank was negligent in following its screening procedures. Privacy rights were again the focus in this case. The court observed that "the donor has a privacy interest in remaining anonymous and avoiding the embarrassment and potential humiliation of being identified as an AIDS carrier." In addition, the societal interest in maintaining an adequate supply of volunteer blood was considered. Unlike the *Rasmussen* court, however, the *Belle Bonfils* court also considered the societal interest in maintaining a safe blood supply. This balancing led to the tailoring of the discovery order in a way that accommodated all competing interests to the extent that was possible.

A final AIDS case dealing with a constitutional right to privacy involved prisoners' constitutional right to privacy regarding their HIV status. In *Woods v. White* (1988), a state prisoner alleged that medical personnel disclosed to nonmedical staff the fact that he had tested positive for HIV. The court cited *Whalen v. Roe* and noted the subsequent consensus among most courts that a right to privacy exists with regard to certain types of personal information. Of particular interest to AIDS researchers is the following observation by the court: "Given the most publicized aspect of the AIDS disease, namely that it is related more closely than most diseases to sexual activity and intravenous drug use, it is difficult to argue that information about this disease is not information of the most personal kind, or that an individual would not have an interest in protecting against the dissemination of such information. . . . I find that plaintiff has a constitutional right to privacy in his medical records" (p. 876).

Taken together, these cases lend strong support to the claim by AIDS research participants that they have a constitutional privacy right that safeguards against forced disclosure of data. Although the balancing of interests involved in each case is and should be unique, surely research participants are entitled in most cases to the same constitutional rights afforded prisoners and blood donors. Thus, several constitutional arguments and supporting cases may be offered to challenge a subpoena for AIDS research data. Even when recognized constitutional rights are involved, however, issues are decided using a case-by-case method, balancing the individual's right to confidentiality against the governmental interest in limited disclosure.

Whatever the merits of a researcher-participant privilege generally, it is clear that the public's interest in the promotion of research on AIDS and participants' interest in privacy may be undermined seriously when protection depends on case-by-case adjudication of these interests. Nevertheless, judicial balancing tests are a common method for resolving disclosure disputes. Fortunately, when judicial protection of ostensibly private research information is sought, researchers need not rely exclusively on constitutional arguments. Privileges that have been recognized under common law and judicial rules that have evolved over the years may also be invoked by way of protecting researchers against compelled disclosures.

Common Law Privileges

As has been discussed at some length, the constitutional arguments for a researcher-participant privilege have not been sufficiently compelling, standing alone, to provide for consistent recognition of the privilege. A somewhat more viable approach may be to rely on the common law privilege, as codified in the Federal Rules of Evidence (Fed. R. Evid.). Rule 501 was enacted in 1975 and states in part: "Except as otherwise required by the Constitution of the United States or provided by Act of Congress or in rules prescribed by the Supreme Court pursuant to statutory authority, the privilege of a witness, person, government, State, or political subdivision thereof shall be governed by the principles of the common law as they may be interpreted by the courts of the United States in the light of reason and experience."

The Supreme Court in *Trammel v. U.S.* (1980, p. 47) held that, by enacting Rule 501, Congress "manifested an affirmative intention not to freeze the law of privilege." Courts are free, therefore, to develop rules of privilege on a case-by-case basis. The privileges recognized by common law included confidential communications between attorney and client, priest and penitent, husband and wife, and psychotherapist and patient. Under common law the communications between doctor and patient were not privileged (e.g., *Whalen v. Roe,* 1977). The recognition of these various privileges is predicated on the belief that individuals would not communicate openly and/or seek services unless the privilege existed. It followed that individuals in need of medical treatment would seek out such treatment regardless of the existence of a doctor-patient privilege (Brown, 1983; Wigmore, 1961).

This reasoning, however, seemingly leads to inconsistent results when applied to those communications to which the privilege does apply. For example, it seems unlikely that people would cease to marry simply because spousal communications were not privileged. Similarly, it is improbable that one in need of the services of an attorney would forego those services merely because the communication was not privileged. Finally, those persons in need of spiritual or other guidance would likely seek the services of a member of the clergy or a mental health professional despite the absence of protection against disclosure.

Thus, when the rationale underlying these common law privileges is applied in different contexts, inconsistent results follow. It seems reasonable to assume that people will be more open in their communications if they can be assured that their communications will not be used against them. However, application of this reasoning to the different relationships presupposes one important fact—that the party knows the privilege exists. Whether individuals are generally aware of the privileged status of their communications is not clear. It may be the case that individuals are more constrained in their communications with others if those communications are not privileged, but those individuals would have to be aware of the privilege to be open in their communications or, alternatively, aware of the absence of the privilege to be more constrained in their communications.

The genesis of these privileges provides some insight. These privileges are more the product of historical precedent than logic. Nevertheless, the rationale underlying the privileges seems particularly applicable to AIDS research participation. In that context, individual participants have much to lose and little to gain by answering personal questions relating to AIDS. Moreover, it seems as though individuals would be deterred from participation in such studies absent an assurance of confidentiality.

Because the interests involved in AIDS research participation so closely parallel the interests involved in other endeavors for which a privilege exists, it is not surprising that many researchers expect courts to protect confidential communication between themselves and their participants. Researchers holding such expectations should be aware of precisely what they are expecting of the courts. In their expectation of such a privilege, researchers are asking that the information obtained from research participants be excluded from the evidentiary fact-finding process engaged in by the judiciary. Because such exclusion frustrates the courts' mission, courts traditionally have been loath to expand the category of communications which are privileged. Yet, in rare instances, the judiciary has recognized certain privileged relationships on its own authority (i.e., without legislative command). In determining whether to create a privilege, the courts must weigh the professional obligation of the social scientist to the research participants against the duty of all citizens, including social scientists, to participate in the fact-finding process.

Evidentiary privileges undermine the principle that every person is obliged to provide all relevant evidence in his or her possession upon subpoena. Thus, unfortunately, researchers can expect little sympathy from courts when asserting a common law right to an evidentiary privilege (Boruch & Cecil, 1979).

When such a privilege has been recognized the practice has been to rely on Dean Wigmore's (1961) four-pronged test:

1. The communication must have originated in a confidential relationship.
2. The preservation of confidentiality must be necessary for the full and satisfactory maintenance of the relationship.
3. The relationship must be one that is important to the community.
4. The injury to the relationship that would accrue from a breach of con-

fidentiality must be greater than the benefit that would be gained for the correct disposal of the litigation.

Despite the courts' reluctance to recognize a broad researcher-participant privilege, most of AIDS research should be able to meet the Wigmore test criteria. The first prong of the test, like "privacy expectation" requirements for a constitutional right to privacy, is circular. One must demonstrate that the relationship is confidential before being granted a common law privilege for confidentiality of the communication. However, participants generally do expect and are promised confidentiality (but see, e.g., Boruch & Cecil, 1979; Stanley, 1987). Furthermore, often AIDS researchers are also in a physician-patient or therapist-client relationship with participants. The confidential nature of the relationship, thus, is more profound.

Ironically, informed consent procedures that clarify potential threats to confidentiality actually may undermine the research participant's expectation of privacy and, therefore, the likelihood that a court would find that a privilege exists. In view, however, of the sensitive nature of research on AIDS and the potential harm that may result from disclosure of records in such research, participants may still reasonably expect maintenance of privacy.

The second Wigmore criterion is also met generally by AIDS researchers. The preservation of confidentiality is necessary for the full and satisfactory maintenance of the relationship in that such a pledge typically is necessary for the recruitment of participants and the receipt of candid responses in AIDS research.

That AIDS research meets the third prong of the test should be self-evident. The importance of research on AIDS to the public health is clear. The terminal nature of the disease, the fear and concern it generates, the fact that expedited reviews of research findings are commonplace, the presentations of summaries of such findings in the mass media, and federal funding of AIDS research all underscore its importance to the community.

The final Wigmore criterion is more problematic simply because it is less predictable. The balancing test involved is necessarily case-specific and depends on trial judge discretion. Although it is difficult to imagine many scenarios in which the balance would not tip toward protection of confidentiality, the range of potential needs for the research data as evidence is sufficiently great as to limit the ability to predict confidently the reliability of Rule 501 in creating a common law privilege. No case has found expressly that a common law researcher-participant privilege exists, and one court has held explicitly that such a privilege does not exist.

In *Wright v. Jeep Corp.* (1982), the defendant in a personal injury action appealed a magistrate's order quashing a subpoena duces tecum to a nonparty expert, a vehicle crash researcher. The court's unwillingness to extend the privilege was explained as follows: "Privileges are the exception to the general duty of every citizen to provide evidence when necessary to further the system of justice. . . . Exceptions to the demand for every man's evidence are not lightly created or expansively construed. . . . This court is unwilling to create a new privilege that would shield academics from testifying" (p. 875).

Thus the prospects for researchers seeking a common law privilege are not good. The research must be deemed confidential, despite the circular definition of confidentiality adopted by the courts, and the interests that militate against disclosure must outweigh those that favor it. Perhaps most importantly, the researcher must find a court that is sympathetic to the common law privilege argument—an argument that no court has accepted. All of this suggests that researchers should look elsewhere for additional, if not alternative, protection.

Federal Rule Protection

Discovery under the Federal Rules. If no statutory, constitutional, or common law privilege is applied to an AIDS researcher's efforts to resist a subpoena, there are additional mechanisms contained in the Federal Rules of Civil Procedure (Fed. R. Civ. P., hereafter Civil Rules) that may afford protection. Section 26(a) lists the following discovery methods: "depositions upon oral examination or written questions; written interrogatories; production of documents or things or permission to enter upon land or other property, for inspection and other purposes; physical and mental examinations; and requests for admission" (Civil Rules, 1991).

Section 26(b) defines the scope and limits of discovery:

(1) Parties may obtain discovery regarding any matter, not privileged, which is relevant to the subject matter involved in the pending action, whether it relates to the claim or defense of the party seeking discovery or to the claim or defense of any other party, including the existence, description, nature, custody, condition and location of any books, documents, or other tangible things and the identity and location of persons having knowledge of any discoverable matter. It is not ground for objection that the information sought will be inadmissible at the trial if the infor-

mation sought appears reasonably calculated to lead to the discovery of admissible evidence. (Civil Rules, 1991)

Quashing or Modifying Subpoenas. Rule 45(a)(1)(C) of the Federal Rules of Civil Procedure and Rule 17(c) of the Federal Rules of Criminal Procedure (Fed. R. Crim. P.) for the United States District Courts (hereafter Criminal Rules), address the scope of subpoenas in adjudicative settings. These rules provide that a subpoena can be used to force production of documentary evidence (i.e., documents, books, or other tangible items) from a person regardless of whether that person is a party to the action involved. However, under Civil Rule 45(c)(3)(B), a court may quash or modify the subpoena if the subpoena:

(i) requires disclosure of a trade secret or other confidential research, development, or commercial information, or

(ii) requires disclosure of an unretained expert's opinion or information not describing specific events or occurrences in dispute and resulting from the expert's study made not at the request of any party.

The Criminal Rules have similar provisions for modification of subpoenas if compliance would be unreasonable or oppressive.

It is worth noting that Civil Rule 45 was recently changed in a manner that may be of particular significance to AIDS researchers. Before December 1991, the language of Civil Rule 45 provided for modification of subpoenas if compliance would be "unreasonable and oppressive." The new language appears to be tailored more narrowly in ways that may meet the needs of researchers seeking to preserve the confidentiality of their research data. Specifically, the language of Rule 45(c)(3)(B)(i), providing for quashing or modifying subpoenas if "confidential research" is at issue, seems promising.

The discovery of information from AIDS researchers may take any of the various forms outlined in Rule 26(a). The scope of discovery is limited by conditions set forth in Rule 26(c), including the availability of protective orders. Compelled disclosure may be denied or modified if a subpoena is found to be unreasonable and oppressive under the Criminal Rules or if it can be included in the categories set forth in Civil Rule 45(c)(3)(B)(i) (e.g., disclosure of a trade secret or confidential information) or 45(c)(3)(B)(ii) (e.g., extraction of expert testimony without compensation). Because these rules apply to federal courts, their use and interpretation are found in court decisions, which vary greatly in some cases. We will discuss several cases that relate to AIDS research and clarify the use of the Federal Rules protections. Although constitutional rights, common law privileges, and Federal Rule protections may all be discussed within one case, we will focus on the Federal Rule at issue and those factors noted in the decisions that are especially relevant.

Pursuant to the protections against subpoenas offered in Rule 45(c) (3)(A), courts may quash or modify a subpoena on grounds of unreasonableness or privilege. Before the enactment of the 1991 rules, the test for modification or quashing of subpoenas was whether they were unreasonable or oppressive. Considerable case law developed around that test, and those decisions are likely to inform rulings on motions to quash or modify under the new rule. Consequently, analysis of the former test and relevant cases follow.

Case Law. Courts typically have employed a three-step analysis, including a balancing of the ascertained interests, to determine whether a judicial subpoena is unreasonable and oppressive (Matherne, 1984). First, the court must determine that the requested information is relevant to the case at hand. Information is relevant if it is "reasonably calculated to lead to the discovery of admissible evidence" (Civil Rules 26[b][1]). If the researcher can convince the court that the subpoenaed information is not relevant to the legal proceeding at hand, the information would not have to be disclosed; however, this criterion is usually met. In addition, once the relevance of the requested material is established, the burden is on the person or party resisting discovery to show "good cause" for nondisclosure or the entry of a protective order (e.g., *Kennedy v. Connecticut Department of Public Safety,* 1987). Once the court has established that the subpoenaed information is relevant, the court must analyze the requesting party's need for the information.

To ascertain need, the court must first determine the importance of the information to the requesting party. Courts use different tests to decide whether information is important. One court, for example, held that the requesting party must demonstrate a "particularized need" (*EEOC v. University of Notre Dame Du Lac,* 1983). Another court created a mathematical formula and defined need as "a function of the probative value of the evidence [which the requesting party] hopes to discover multiplied by the likelihood that it will be discovered as a result of the instant subpoena" (*Andrews v. Eli Lilly & Co.,* 1983, p. 498 n.12).

Regardless of the particular test employed by the court, if it finds that the information is crucial to the requesting party's case, the court generally will order disclosure of the information. Conversely, when the subpoenaed documents are of questionable importance to the requesting party's case, the court examines the party's need for the information more critically and is less likely to force disclosure of the subpoenaed material. If a party fails to demonstrate convincingly a need for the requested information, the court will not enforce the subpoena if there are countervailing reasons for nondisclosure.

Kennedy v. Conn. Dept. of Public Safety (1987) demonstrates a situation wherein a request for information is crucial to the requesting party's case. Kennedy was a civil rights, sexual discrimination case, in which plaintiffs alleged a violation of Title VII of the Civil Rights Act by the State of Connecticut (Title VII prohibits harassment in the workplace). In the court's determination of the plaintiff's need for information from a nonparty who was conducting academic research at the time and place the discriminatory conduct allegedly occurred, they noted that society, and the plaintiff, have an extraordinarily important interest in ensuring that civil rights are respected. "If [the researcher] actually witnessed such critical facts, any first hand information she possesses would relate directly to the merits of the case, hold the potential of equally benefiting each side to the lawsuit, and provide valuable assistance to the trier of fact in its search for the truth" (p. 499). The court then distinguished circumstances that involve eyewitness knowledge, that require testimony, and information regarding scholarly conclusions, academic opinions, and occurrences reportedly conveyed in "confidence" by nonparty research subjects. The court's discussion of this "other" requested information in *Kennedy* is of particular interest for an evaluation of AIDS researchers' confidentiality protections. In this case, the nonparty researcher had stated in the informed consent forms: "under no circumstances will the facts observed, or the opinions held by the P.I. [principal investigator] be revealed to any other party" (Exhibit D, page 4) (p. 498). Also a model informed consent form indicated that the research project constituted a "privileged relationship" and that "confidentiality and anonymity are guaranteed" (p. 498).

The court was not persuaded by her unfounded claims to a privileged relationship. Nevertheless, the court respected the legitimate concern that O'Connell (the researcher) was a scholar who obtained certain information under a promise of confidentiality, and that requiring her to divulge the identities of those individuals who communicated with her under such a promise conceivably could jeopardize an important scholar-subject trust relationship without clearly serving a transcendent interest. Therefore, without abrogation of the plaintiff's right to apply to the court at a later date if necessary, the court held that O'Connell could delete, at her own expense, from the documents that she produced the names of individuals whose communications to her assertedly were given under a promise of confidentiality. Thus, even though the claimed researcher privilege was legally unsubstantiated in this case, the court recognized the importance of such relationships and the need for continued research enterprises unhampered by unnecessary disclosures, while allowing for further disclosure if the plaintiff could at a later date show compelling need for it.

A second set of issues that the court confronts when determining whether the requesting party needs the subpoenaed information is the likelihood that the requesting party can get the information from another source (*In re Dinnan,* 1981) or that disclosure of documents would require a duplication of effort (*Tavoulareas v. Piro,* 1981). In these situations, even if the requesting party adequately demonstrates compelling need for the information, the court is unlikely to force disclosure from the subpoenaed person (see *Carl Zeisa Stiftung v. V.E.B. Carl Zeiss,* 1966; *Eglin Fed. Credit Union v. Cantor, Fitzgerald Sec. Corp.,* 1981; *In re Penn Central Commercial Paper Litigation,* 1973; *Ohio-Sealy Mattress Mfg. Co. v. Sealy, Inc.,* 1981).

For example, in *Apicella v. McNeil Laboratories, Inc.* (1975), the court declined to compel disclosure in part because the parties to the action had failed to show that the information requested was not available through other sources. In that case, a patient who suffered permanent disabilities after receiving a drug brought an action against the manufacturer. The manufacturer and the patient sought an order to compel a third-party publisher of a medical newsletter (which contained an article on deaths allegedly related to the drug the patient had received) to disclose the name of the person who wrote the original draft and to produce related correspondence. Of interest to AIDS researchers (who may provide information for publication anonymously) is the court's additional consideration in its denial of an order to disclose that such an order might seriously affect the ability of a publisher to obtain information from those (in this case physicians) who wished to remain anonymous in the future.

Once the court has determined that the subpoenaed material is relevant and the requesting party needs the information, the court must consider the burden that enforcement of the subpoena would impose. The burdensomeness test finds its genesis in the Fourth Amendment, which prescribes that disclosure shall not be unreasonable (*Oklahoma Press Publishing Co. v. Walling,* 1946). Whether a disclosure is unduly burdensome depends on the particular facts of each case, and no hard and fast rule can be applied to resolve the question (*F.T.C. v. Shaffner,* 1980). However, there are several factors that courts generally consider in determining burdensomeness—the breadth and specificity of the request, the subpoenaed party's ability to incur expenses, the time period that the request covers, and the reasons underlying the request (Matherne, 1984).

Courts may not enforce a subpoena if the request for information is not defined with sufficient specificity, or a specific request's breadth would place an unnecessary burden on the subpoenaed party. The subpoenaed person must endure some degree of hardship. A claim of inconvenience, for example, would not frustrate a proper request for information (see *Freeman v. Seligson,* 1968; *Westinghouse Elec. Corp. v. City of Burlington,* 1965). Related to the consideration of breadth is the time period covered by the request. Courts may not enforce a subpoena that spans an unreasonable time period (see *United States v. IBM,* 1975).

Furthermore, although the person subject to a request for information must absorb some degree of expense in producing the documents, the cost must be reasonable. To determine the reasonableness of cost, the court examines the relative size and resources of the parties (see *Celanese Corp. v. E. I. duPont de Nemours & Co.,* 1973). The court then determines whether the expense should be borne by the requesting party or the subpoenaed party. If the requesting party has meager resources and the subpoenaed party has vast resources, the subpoenaed party could be instructed to bear the cost of production (see *Blank v. Talley Indus., Inc.,* 1972). Because the new rules authorize attorneys to issue subpoenas (as opposed to courts under the old rules), there is some concern that adverse counsel will not take seriously the costs of production. The new Rules 45(c)(1) address this issue as follows: "A party or an attorney responsible for the issuance and service of a subpoena shall take reasonable steps to avoid imposing undue burden or expense on a person subject to that subpoena. The court on behalf of which the subpoena was issued shall enforce this duty and impose upon the party or attorney in breach of this duty an appropriate sanction, which may include, but is not limited to, lost earnings and a reasonable attorney's fee."

Finally, in determining burdensomeness, the court may consider the purpose of the information request. This issue relates to need in that a legitimate need would favor disclosure, and a conjectural or speculative need would not favor disclosure (see *Andrews v. Eli Lilly & Co.*, 1983). In addition, the court would deny the request if made in bad faith (Matherne, 1984). The Federal Rules controlling discovery contemplate an exercise of good faith in all discovery requests (*Georgia Power Co. v. EEOC*, 1968). If bad faith exists, the discovery request violates federal discovery procedures and thus is unenforceable (see *H. Kessler & Co. v. EEOC*, 1971).

In re Snyder (1987) was a case involving a burdensome subpoena where the court recognized potential situations for using the court system in bad faith. The case involved an action for personal injuries sustained in a motor vehicle accident. The defendant manufacturer obtained a subpoena duces tecum against a nonparty researcher who was the author of a report on the safety of motor vehicles. The researcher moved to quash the subpoena. The District Court held that the subpoena was excessively burdensome, given the amount of information sought, the collateral relationship of the report to the action, and the fact that the manufacturer (American Motors Corporation [AMC]) had sought the researcher's account of this study through similar subpoenas on at least three separate occasions in different cases.

In 1982, the District Court for the Eastern District of Michigan refused to quash a similar subpoena brought by Jeep Corporation in another personal injury action (*Wright v. Jeep Corp.*, 1982). In this case the District Court held that the researcher had no privilege not to testify, and, as material sought was relevant to the lawsuit, his testimony would be compelled. The court reasoned that no confidentiality had been demonstrated, and the possibility of being subpoenaed would not chill writers and researchers sufficiently to warrant a special exemption from their duty to provide evidence.

Shortly after the *Wright* decision, the Sixth Circuit upheld another decision from the Eastern District of Michigan (*Buchanan v. American Motors Corp.*, 1983), this one quashing AMC's subpoena of Snyder (the researcher) in a product's liability suit, on the ground of burdensomeness. The court stated that it would require a nonparty to spend a large amount of time compiling numerous files, and a compelling justification of need was not demonstrated.

The *Buchanan* court noted that AMC's series of demands of Snyder, who was a stranger to each of the lawsuits, sufficed to establish the excessively burdensome nature of AMC's discovery efforts. The court made note of the legal expense and personal disruption prompted by the discovery efforts and observed that Snyder had retired. The court, observing that the subpoenas were both qualitatively and quantitatively burdensome, stated the opinion that "at some point, even a subpoena of modest scope will likely be quashed because it will be one too many" (p. 214).

The court then chronicled some of the problems inherent in the subpoena process as follows: "Discovery offers an avenue for indirect harassment of researchers whose published work points to defects in products or practices. There exists also a potential for harassment of members of the public who volunteer, under a promise of confidentiality, to provide information for use in such studies" (p. 216). The *Buchanan* court concluded by recognizing that scientific and applied research is valuable to society and calls for changes that will facilitate the continuation of relatively unhampered research.

The new Rules have addressed one aspect of the problems presented by cases like *Buchanan*. Rule 45(c)(3)(B)(ii) addresses those cases wherein subpoenas "require . . . disclosure of an unretained expert's opinion or information not describing specific events or occurrences in dispute and resulting from the expert's study made not at the request of any party." Unfortunately for AIDS researchers, the rule does not provide for modifying or quashing subpoenas, but merely authorizes courts to make them conditional on "assur[ances] that the person to whom the subpoena is addressed will be reasonably compensated" (Civil Rules 45(c)(3)(B)(iii)). The interests sought to be protected by this rule, thus, are not concerned with confidentiality but rather with economics. One author has observed that the clause "seeks to guard against anything that can amount to an expert opinion from that person if no compensation has been arranged for it" (Siegel, 1992, p. 234).

It is clear that no single factor is conclusive evidence of unreasonableness and oppression. Courts must weigh all elements to determine whether the burden of a subpoena on a researcher is excessive and should be quashed or modified. So far we have addressed only one of the mechanisms available from federal civil procedure rules for protecting information from subpoenas. Quashing a subpoena on the ground of unreasonableness occurs only when absolutely necessary. More often, after the court has balanced the interests involved, it will modify a subpoena or grant a protective order so that some disclosure of information will be allowed. In addition, there is another section of the Civil Rules that provides further grounds for protection of requested research information.

Protective Orders

Section 26 of the Civil Rules covers the general provisions for discovery in federal courts. Although section 26(c) in many ways is redundant with section 45(b), it does provide for additional protection conditions and provides several different protective orders that a court may grant to reduce the burden that a subpoena imposes on the subpoenaed party. Rule 26(c) allows for the imposition of protective conditions upon a showing of "embarrassment, oppression, or undue burden or expense." Of primary concern to AIDS researchers is the Rule's provision for protection to guard against embarrassment.

A protective order is a device that the court authorizes and constructs to allow discovery subject to various degrees of limitation. The purpose of a protective measure is to temper the expansive scope of discovery and to protect individuals who become involved in the discovery process, whether voluntarily or involuntarily. Rule 26(c) provides eight protective measures, and courts may establish additional means of protection as justice requires. The eight specified measures allow courts to order:

1. That the discovery not be had;
2. That the discovery may be had only on specified terms and conditions, including a designation of the time or place;
3. That the discovery may be had only by a method of discovery other than that selected by the party seeking discovery;
4. That certain matters not be inquired into, or that the scope of the discovery be limited to certain matters;
5. That discovery be conducted with no one present except persons designated by the court;
6. That a deposition after being sealed be opened only by order of the court;
7. That a trade secret or other confidential research, development, or commercial information not be disclosed or be disclosed only in a designated way and;
8. That the parties simultaneously file specified documents or information enclosed in sealed envelopes to be opened as directed by the court.

There are several court decisions that have used these procedural mechanisms for resolving disputes involving researchers and their attempts to quash subpoenas for their research data.

Case Law. Andrews v. Eli Lilly & Co. (1983) was decided according to former rule 45(b) and rule 26(c). The court noted that in determining whether persons who seek to have a subpoena quashed have met their burden of showing unreasonableness or oppression, courts must balance the hardship imposed by quashing the subpoena against the hardship imposed on such persons by permitting the discovery. This case is often cited by researchers as the precedent for quashing subpoenas on the grounds that disclosure of confidential information would jeopardize research projects. In addition, the text of the opinion is rife with language alluding to the importance of research and the potential dangers inherent in disclosure of "confidential" research, particularly premature disclosure of information.

Andrews involved a motion to quash a subpoena in which the manufacturer of diethylstilbestrol (DES) sought production of records relating to a research project identifying the correlation between DES use by pregnant women and the later development of adenocarcinoma of the vagina in their female offspring. The court quashed the subpoena of nonparty research data because the manufacturer's need for such evidence was speculative and uncertain, and its interest in defending itself was outweighed by the danger that the disclosure of confidential information would jeopardize the research project and similar projects. Additionally, it was not shown that deletion of names from the records would prevent breach of confidentiality. The court noted that there is undoubtedly a compelling social interest in promoting research. If the registry were destroyed, a unique and vital resource for learning about the incidence, causes, and treatment of adenocarcinoma would be lost; thus, a First Amendment free flow of information interest was at stake.

The court extensively cited material from affidavits given by experts. The dangers of premature disclosure of research data were considered.

> Disclosure of information from ongoing epidemiological research can seriously undermine the study since premature disclosure of information, before valid conclusions can be reached by the researchers, may suggest faulty conclusions. These in turn may improperly discredit the study. On the other hand, given an opportunity to complete the research unobstructed by disclosure request[s], would have the greatest likelihood of achieving tested and supported conclusions. Any forced premature disclosure could subject the researchers to professional ridicule and criticism. (Affidavit of Leonard T. Kurland, *Andrews*, pp. 502–503)

The court also noted that disclosure of tentative analyses of data and drafts of articles can adversely impact the exchange of ideas relating to ongoing research.

> Epidemiological investigators, and indeed medical investigators in general, pursuing the spirit of scientific inquiry, often speculate, hypothesize and draw possible and probable conclusions as they probe various questions related to their research. Freedom to proceed in this manner requires confidentiality. Involuntary disclosure of this uninhibited communication among scientists to parties that are not participants in the research demolishes the freedom of thought and interchange of ideas that is so essential to productive research. Also, interpretation of the speculations, hypotheses, and possible or probable conclusions by outsiders carries a serious risk of being faulty, resulting in medical misinformation and possibly unjustifiably discrediting the investigators. (Affidavit of Robert E. Scully, *Andrews*, p. 503)

Despite this case's important holdings and its potential utility as precedent, it was reversed on appeal in *Deitchman v. E. R. Squibb & Sons, Inc.* (1984). A court's decision to quash is reversible on appeal only for abuse of discretion by the trial court. Because the trial judge has wide latitude in controlling matters of discovery, appellate courts rarely find an abuse of discretion. Nevertheless, the appellate court in this case found that to give Squibb virtually no information at all was an abuse of discretion.

Fortunately, the court's reversal was not altogether adverse to the lower court's findings. Their reversal focused on the court's duty when confronted with a motion to quash a subpoena. The appellate court stated that a court's duty is not to deny any discovery but to reduce the demand to what is reasonable, considering the discoverer's needs and the discoveree's interests. Thus, the *Deitchman* court vacated and remanded the case to the District court, directing it to exercise its discretion with sufficient flexibility to allow defendant Squibb the discovery that was necessary in the circumstances without doing harm needlessly to the legitimate concerns of the subpoenaed registry. The appellate court noted that, although they do not believe that this case calls for release of identifying information, nonidentifying information should be provided to Squibb.

Of interest to AIDS researchers is the additional case information included in the appellate court's opinion. The court revealed that the university registry subpoenaed was the only centralized repository of information for the disease of clear cell adenocarcinoma of the genital tract. To establish the registry, Dr. Herbst sent letters of inquiry to all departments of medical schools in the United States, to hospitals throughout the world that specialize in cancer treatment, and to the World Health Organization. He promised that the registry would keep confidential all information submitted to it.

The court was respectful of these promises but stated that where substantial need is shown, the release of even confidential matter may be compelled. In contrast to the *Andrews* court, the appellate court found that for Squibb to be able to prepare a proper defense, access to the registry data was absolutely essential. They believed that it was possible to have fashioned a protective order or modified the subpoena in some way so as to protect the registry against any loss of confidential information, while still giving Squibb discoverable information.

These two cases demonstrate the unreliability of the balancing test provided by the Civil Rules. Although ultimately "confidential" information is protected, the scope of the protection and the particular factors that were balanced differed for these courts. It is clear from these cases that even if all the factors to be considered by a court were known, the court's ultimate decision would remain something of a mystery for predictive purposes. The cases that follow do little to clear up this mystery but do address issues that relate more directly to AIDS research.

In *Lampshire v. Procter & Gamble Co.* (1982), the Centers for Disease Control (CDC) filed a motion for a protective order pursuant to 26(c) seeking to prevent a tampon manufacturer from obtaining discovery of personal identifying information about women involved in its study of toxic shock syndrome (TSS), in connection with a products liability suit against the tampon manufacturer seeking redress for injuries allegedly resulting from TSS. The court held that the manufacturer's need for the information was insufficient to justify intrusion on participants' privacy. The court noted that nothing in Rule 26(c) suggests that the availability of a protective order hinges on the existence of a privilege. The rule allows a protective order to be entered upon a simple showing of good cause by the movant (party that moves [i.e., makes the motion]). The court stated its opinion that: "The information obtained by the CDC from its subjects in the studies on TSS is quite personal and sensitive. It is imminently appropriate to protect the subjects of the CDC studies, who may have no connection with this lawsuit, from questions by strangers about such personal matters" (p. 60).

The "personal and sensitive" nature of AIDS research is likely to equal, if not surpass, the "personal and sensitive" nature of TSS research. AIDS research participants are probably as estranged from the parties seeking discovery as those in TSS research. The implications of this holding for AIDS researchers are both clear and encouraging.

Farnsworth v. Procter and Gamble Co. (1985) presented another set of cases against Procter and Gamble in a products liability action for injuries suffered from TSS. It too involved a subpoena for CDC's research information. The lower court granted a protective order to the CDC that prevented Procter and Gamble from gaining access to the names and addresses of the women in the studies. The case was appealed to the Court of Appeals for the Eleventh Circuit. The higher court began by admitting that the American legal system and the specific rules of the federal courts strongly favor full discovery whenever possible; the law's basic presumption is that the public is entitled to every person's evidence. However, despite these factors supporting a grant of access to the evidence, the higher court upheld the district court's protective order for essentially the same reasons as those described in *Andrews*. The appellate court focused on the compelling social interest in promoting research and the potential future harm to CDC's public health mission if information were released:

> The Center's purpose is the protection of the public's health. Central to this purpose is the ability to conduct probing scientific and social research supported by a population willing to submit to in-depth questioning. Undisputed testimony in the record indicates that disclosure of the names and addresses of these research participants could seriously damage this voluntary reporting. Even without an express guarantee of confidentiality there is still an expectation, not unjustified, that when highly personal and potentially embarrassing information is given for the sake of medical research, it will remain private. (p. 1547)

The CDC's victories in these cases should be viewed as welcome by AIDS researchers. Like efforts by the CDC, AIDS researchers' efforts are largely dependent on "a population willing to submit to in-depth questioning." The court's willingness to protect potentially embarrassing, highly personal information in TSS cases may have beneficial consequences for AIDS researchers seeking protection against disclosure of research data.

Finally, in *Richards of Rockford, Inc. v. Pacific Gas & Elec.* (1976), the court also focused on the need for confidentiality in research. It found that the requested information was largely supplementary and held that, as such, the balance was weighted toward nondisclosure. The motion to compel a third-party researcher to produce documents was denied. The case involved a breach of contract and defamation action in which the plaintiff sought to compel a third-party research assistant for a university professor to testify and to produce documents concerning confidential interviews with employees of the defendant. The court noted that counsel produced an impressive series of affidavits from scholars throughout the country attesting to the necessity of maintaining confidential relationships for the accomplishment of their research. From this, the court concluded: "Much of the raw data on which research is based simply is not made available except upon a pledge of confidentiality. Compelled disclosure of confidential information would without question severely stifle research into questions of public policy, the very subjects in which the public interest is greatest" (p. 390).

This case is important to AIDS researchers because it is what might be characterized as a "pure research" justification for protection against subpoenas. The cases mentioned previously were concerned with very sensitive questions relating to disease and other personal matters. Although AIDS research certainly would qualify as being under the same rubric, *Richards* seems to stand for the proposition that the continued conduct of research, in and of itself, justifies some limiting of discovery procedures.

Comment on the New Federal Rule 45

As has been mentioned, Rule 45 has been changed recently in ways that might affect AIDS researchers. Because of the relative novelty of these changes, no substantive, dispositive case law has been developed. Nevertheless, a few features of the new rule warrant at least some attention.

A fairly significant change in Rule 45 now authorizes attorneys to issue subpoenas. Under the former rule, only courts could do so. This is likely to have little impact, however, because the practice for some years has been for courts to issue subpoenas practically "in blank," allowing the requesting attorney to define the contours of the order. Although this might seem to be problematic at first, some reigning in of adverse counsel is provided for by Rule 45(c)(1). This issue is discussed in greater detail in the Case Law subsection of the Quashing or Modifying Subpoenas section above.

Also Rule 45 now provides for a simple duces tecum subpoena of information and materials possessed by nonparties. Previously, the acquisition of materials must have been made in conjunction with a deposition or trial. The risks of premature or uninformed disclosure of research data have been discussed elsewhere in this volume. The significance of this change for AIDS researchers is that the new rule allows the party issuing the subpoena to get materials with no explanation from the researcher; thus, the opportunity to address misunderstanding or misuse preventively is diminished.

It is also worth noting that Rule 45 allows the subpoenaed party to serve the party issuing the subpoena with written objections to the subpoena. This typically temporarily suspends the servee's obligation to comply and shifts the burden to the issuer to demonstrate why compliance should be ordered. This is often a very tricky procedure—one not to be undertaken without legal advice.

Perhaps the most significant change in Rule 45 is in section (c)(3)(A)(iii). That section now holds that courts (if the motions are timely) "*shall* quash or modify the subpoena if it . . . requires disclosure of privileged or other protected matter and no exception or waiver applies" (emphasis added). Although such power has always existed implicitly, explicit reference to privileged information in Rule 45 may indicate an increased willingness to protect that information from subpoenas. Because these changes are fairly new, however, it is too early to tell what impact they will have.

Administrative Protection of Confidentiality

In addition to direct legal protection for research confidentiality (i.e., statutory, judicial), the legal system, through administrative procedures, may protect the confidentiality of research participants by placing constraints on researchers' "voluntary disclosures" of confidential research information. Such "voluntary" disclosures, that is, disclosures that are not compelled from any outside authority, may occur because of conflicting demands that have been placed on the researcher for disclosure (e.g., reporting a person's health status to protect another from exposure, even though not obligated through any duty to protect or other legal obligation), ignorance (e.g., compliance with a disclosure request without questioning its authority or realizing that a challenge could be successful), or carelessness (reporting results in such a way that deductive disclosure of information occurs). Unfortunately, "voluntary" disclosures may also occur intentionally because of a lack of professionalism (e.g., telling family and friends their participants' names and other confidential information).

Institutional Review Boards (IRBs) are one type of administrative body that may provide some protection against such disclosures. Proposals for research on AIDS almost invariably involve more than minimal risk to participants and should be accorded full IRB review before implementation

(Bayer et al., 1984). IRBs, in turn, probably will find it useful to consult with affected groups (Committee for the Protection of Human Participants in Research [CPHPR], 1985; Office for Protection from Research Risks [OPRR], 1984).

Funding agencies may also help curtail inappropriate, unnecessary, or excessive disclosures. When federal funding is requested, peer reviewers and agency officers carefully scrutinize the ethical implications of the research. This high standard of review should help to ensure that appropriate protections of confidentiality are built into the research design whenever possible (Committee for the Protection of Human Participants in Research, 1982; Office for Protection from Research Risks, 1984) and that privacy is not compromised simply because of investigator carelessness or ignorance.

Review of the adequacy of protections built into a research design, of course, does not guarantee that researchers will exercise appropriate stewardship of the data. However, it is possible for administrative funding agencies to put some "teeth" into their reviews by imposing sanctions on inappropriate behavior. The availability of administrative remedies for unethical conduct may provide effective deterrents. For example, agencies can tailor grant restrictions to the particular ethical issues raised by a project (e.g., the need to protect confidentiality in research on AIDS) and then impose sanctions that impact on researchers' livelihoods on such restrictions. Administrative sanctions may include: (a) termination of the grant; (b) mandatory refund of the grant; (c) suspension of pending future grants; (d) the attachment of a record of the incident to any applications for future grants; and (e) termination of eligibility for grant awards (Greenstein, 1984).

Compelling arguments can be made that all necessary restrictions on research should be imposed through the grant or contract. In this way, the terms for disclosure can be tailored to fit the particular case. Consequently, proscribed and prescribed conduct should be clear to both the researcher and the government. Additionally, the researcher should be better informed about disclosure requirements because the researcher is more likely to read her grant or contract than she is to read the Code of Federal Regulations. However, it is questionable whether such restrictions would be legally binding on courts. Moreover, granting agencies presently do not enforce available sanctions for inappropriate voluntary disclosure.

If administrative controls over researchers' voluntary disclosures are ineffective or nonexistent, sanctions for such disclosures are still available, to a limited degree, through the traditional judicial forums. Three grounds for suits against a researcher for disclosure of confidential data exist. It is worth noting that these grounds are available whether the disclosure was made voluntarily or under a court order. First, the research participant may seek a tort recovery based on a breach by the researcher of a duty not to invade privacy by disclosing confidential information. Whether the disclosure was made pursuant to judicial, legislative, or administrative proceedings, the disclosure is considered privileged and is subject to legal redress. Second, the participant might claim that a contract, including a promise of confidentiality, between the participant and the researcher existed and was breached. Third, a participant may claim that the researcher acquired the sensitive information by a misrepresentation about its confidentiality.

Although researchers may raise the objection that they were forced to disclose on pain of criminal sanction, in fact, such "crimes" are unlikely to apply to researchers. Three possible theories of liability have been proposed: (a) researchers who keep secret evidence of crimes committed by others are accessories to those crimes after the fact; (b) they are guilty of the separate crime of misprision of felony (i.e., concealing knowledge of a felony); or (c) they are guilty of the crime of obstruction of justice.

Despite these possible criminal sanctions for nondisclosure, researchers are unlikely to be prosecuted successfully under any of them. The first sanction probably would not apply to researchers. The most common rule is that mere failure to give information of a crime will not make one an accessory after the fact absent other acts of comfort or assistance (*Levering v. Commonwealth*, 1909). The second sanction is unlikely to have any effect because misprision of felony has been abandoned or is unrecognized in most jurisdictions. The final criminal law for nondisclosures "does not reach silence alone." The essence of an obstruction of justice lies in the commission of acts that impede, rather than in failure to aid, the administration of justice. Thus, although these theories have been advanced as potentially imposing criminal liability for the attempts of researchers to protect participants' confidential information from disclosure, such arguments are, at best, weak.

Conclusion

Researchers have at their disposal a number of potential sources of protection for confidential information acquired during the conduct of research. Participants have at their disposal a number of remedies for breaches of confidentiality, many of which impose sanctions against researchers. Finally, IRBs, funding agencies, and others can play vital roles in ensuring that confidential information remains confidential. All of these can and should be utilized in ways that maximize confidentiality.

Chapter 6

AIDS, FEAR, AND SCIENCE

Private biases may be outside the law, but the law cannot, directly or indirectly, give them effect.

Palmore v. Sidoti

Following our fairly detailed accounts in Chapters 2 through 4 of the kind of balancing of interests that occurs within particular bodies of law, in Chapter 5 we moved up one level of analysis and considered the degree to which other bodies of law may be brought to bear on particular issues. The inquiry cannot end there, however. For better or for worse, decisions will also be influenced by broader concerns, often wholly outside the law.

The law is a social institution that parallels other social institutions. In important ways, it is a microcosm of our society. At times, the law drives society; at other times, society drives the law. Thus, to understand fully the various influences at work in AIDS research, we must abandon the (usually) sterile rationality of the law and turn to the somewhat less rational response of our society to the AIDS crisis.

Fear and Public Policy

The psychological reality of AIDS is that it evokes fear. AIDS is not logical; it is hard to believe that a contagious disease so deadly can be transmitted in such limited ways. As a task force of the American College Health Association observed, it is "no wonder . . . that people are afraid: a new disease, a relatively short period of observation, rapidly increasing numbers of cases, a long clinical incubation period, healthy carriers, and a dreadful outlook" (Keeling, 1986, p. viii). Moreover, the distinction between "sexual behavior causing disease and sexual behavior resulting in effective transmission" is subtle (Valdiserri, 1987, p. 99), although decisions originating in confusion on this point can be profoundly misguided.

Such a set of facts and such an epidemic of fear have ample historical precedent (Brandt, 1988; Cutler & Arnold, 1988; Valdiserri, 1987), but the lack of uniqueness does not attenuate the perniciousness of the social order that fear generates. Although some of the worst examples of discriminatory behavior (e.g., school exclusion) seem to appear with less frequency and the law now makes such attempts less likely (Americans with Disabilities Act of 1990), fearful, mistaken, and sometimes mean-spirited attitudes persist in a substantial segment of the population. About half of American adults say that they would avoid a grocery store if the owner had AIDS, and nearly one-third advocate the quarantine and publication of the names of people with the disease (Herek & Capitanio, in press). Almost half continue to believe that some forms of casual contagion (e.g., a kiss on the cheek) or airborne transmission (e.g., sneezing) can result in HIV infection. One in five African Americans believes that AIDS is the product of a government-sponsored program of genocide, and about four in ten people, regardless of race, believe that information about the disease is being withheld from the public (Herek & Capitanio, in press).

There can be no doubt that hysteria about AIDS has led many policy-makers to support measures that have little, if any, rational basis. A particularly glaring example was the overwhelming vote of the Illinois legislature to reaffirm its action requiring premarital HIV testing, even though in just five months, the "requirement . . . cost marriage applicants up to $250 each, caused hundreds of couples to travel outside the state to wed, and turned up only five HIV+ people out of 30,000 tested" ("Illinois Passes," 1988; cf. Cleary et al., 1987; Hardy, 1991; McKillip, 1991). Still, the bigger message may be that the data ultimately overcame the paranoia, and the law eventually was repealed (see McKillip, 1991).

The Political Context for AIDS Research

Political Constraints on Research

In the sense that political decisions generate the money that supports AIDS research, politics drives the endeavor. However, it also sometimes stops the enterprise. A recent editorial in the *American Journal of Public Health* that urged the "emancipation" of the Centers for Disease Control (Susser, 1993) was illustrative. The point was that the politicization of the CDC had impeded important prevention research and action.

No better example of such deterrence of important work has been the bar on federal support of surveys of adolescent sexual behavior—critical information for development and evaluation of programs to prevent HIV infection among adolescents (see Henggeler et al., 1992, p. 124). Although the topic has not gone completely unstudied (see Taylor, 1993b, describing major British, French, and American surveys about sexual behavior), there is no question that prevention-related research has been slowed substantially.

Indeed, the decision about which research should *not* be supported has often turned on the political acceptability of particular interventions; too often policymakers have been unwilling even to support experiments that, if properly designed, would provide critical data for policy development. For example, American policymakers have generally refused to permit tests of the efficacy of needle-exchange programs despite evidence that (a) many of even the intravenous drug users who are not in treatment have made changes toward safer behavior (see, e.g., "Update: Reducing HIV Transmission," 1990); (b) treatment is insufficiently available; and (c) needle-exchange programs abroad have resulted in safer behavior without an increase in drug use (see Adler, 1992a; Case et al., 1992; Friedman, 1992; Hooker, 1992; Stryker, 1989; Youngstrom, 1992).

Politics has intruded even on scholars' ability to discuss important questions of AIDS policy and law. Notably, publicity about the International Conferences on AIDS has tended to focus on the limits placed on travel by delegates with HIV infections and on the disruptions of key addresses that sometimes have occurred. Similarly, practitioners in the field have quarreled about the number of free passes to the International Conferences that should be provided to people with AIDS (McCusick, 1990).

In the face of constraints on major lines of research, parallel limitations on the design and reporting of research, and public debates about the adequacy of research involving particular populations, researchers may wonder why they did not major in political science. In any event, they are apt to feel unjustly constrained by considerations that have little to do with the risk that people with HIV infections pose or the probable effectiveness of particular prevention or treatment strategies.

Bad Science Makes Bad Policy

The temptation of scientists is to regard many policymakers as people who, whether purposefully or unwittingly, often cater to public fears and who often get in the way of development of the knowledge base needed for rational and humane policy. That view, of course, is not without merit. Nonetheless, it should be remembered that bad science is a particularly efficient means of creation of bad policy. No single event may have been as influential in fomenting fear as was an article on pediatric AIDS by an important clinical researcher (Oleske et al., 1983) that was published with an accompanying editorial in the *Journal of the American Medical Association* and a related news release. That article suggested, contrary to the data, that AIDS could be transmitted by casual contact. The epidemic of fear was started: within a week, San Francisco police and firefighters were wearing gloves and masks (Batchelor, 1988; Shilts, 1987).

The public's fear was intensified later by the publication of Masters, Johnson, and Kolodny's (1988) book purporting to show that experts were "gravely underestimating the degree to which the AIDS virus has spread into the heterosexual community" (p. 4). Because of the notoriety of Masters and Johnson, their report received substantial press attention, and some policymakers turned to means of identifying and controlling heterosexuals with HIV infections. The study that they described had obvious methodological flaws (notably, reliance on convenience samples, including a sample of adults who reported many sexual partners), but their own data failed to support their conclusions (Kaplan, 1988).

Although the motives that underlay these incidents were not clear (perhaps there was simple negligence involved), the likelihood of their occurrence may be heightened by the pressure for quick publication—a phenomenon that may impede deliberative analysis and reporting. In view of the competing interest in speedy application of findings that may facilitate prevention or treatment of AIDS, the Institute of Medicine has advocated establishment of a "mechanism for public reporting of data with clinical urgency soon after trial completion and prior to journal publication" (Institute of Medicine, 1991, p. 13). Although such a procedure would be responsive to the public need for information, it may also leave considerable room for error.

Sometimes Good Science Makes Bad Policy

Even when care is taken, the topic is sufficiently sensitive and the politics sufficiently complex that even careful discussion of ideas may lead to unwarranted consequences. An example that has not yet erupted into highly politicized conflict but that has the potential to do so is the neighborhood focus recently recommended in the National Research Council report on "The Social Impact of AIDS" (discussed by Kolata, 1993). The authors of that report argued for targeted AIDS prevention because of "the pattern of AIDS's spread and the success of programs that have focused tightly on affected groups and neighborhoods" (p. 1). The report suggested that "AIDS is devastating a handful of neighborhoods while leaving most of the nation unscathed" (p. 1). The authors recommended focusing American efforts on explicit AIDS education, needle exchanges, and other approaches matched to neighborhood language and mores.

The idea is a provocative one, well supported by geographic distribution of AIDS cases even within particular cities. Most AIDS cases in New York City, for example, are found in about a half-dozen neighborhoods. Nonetheless, the possibility of misinterpretation of the findings and discriminatory application of them (in effect, development of AIDS ghettos) has to be considered. A California researcher described an earlier similar problem:

> At the University of California at San Francisco, we did our first project in AIDS epidemiology—a study of incidence rates in gay neighborhoods of San Francisco—at the end of 1982, just when the epidemic was coming to public consciousness. We did it by identifying neighborhoods of the city in which large numbers of homosexual men lived. This felt, and still feels, like drawing a wall around the ghetto. It led me and others to be extremely paranoid about publishing the results for fear of providing a target—for example, to insurance companies seeking to redline homosexual neighborhoods. (Moss, 1989, pp. 176–177)

At the same time, researchers may fear giving the "wrong" message, simply because in doing so they risk loss of access to research participants. Bayer (1989) described an example of "laundering" observations to fit the desires of a community on whom researchers were dependent:

> Perhaps most remarkable in the city's well-prepared case [defending an attempt to close the bathhouses in San Francisco] was the failure to obtain a clear declaration of support for closure from any nationally known epidemiologist involved in the study of AIDS and the patterns of sexual behavior among gay men. For [public health officials in San Francisco], it was clear that investigators dependent upon the cooperation of the gay community feared that collaboration with the San Francisco authorities would result in a rupture of professionally critical relationships of trust. (p. 48)

As discussed in Chapter 1, AIDS research is filled with conflicts of interest. Sensitivity to political concerns has the potential both to enhance and to distort the search for knowledge. Thus, researchers on AIDS are often faced with hard choices about the openness with which they describe their observations and analyses. Do they risk alienation of their sources of information or, perhaps worse, unintended ostracism of participant groups when frank discussion of results may lead to either social consequence?

The Evolution of the Law

Beginning with *Palmore v. Sidoti* (1984, quoted at the beginning of this chapter), a case in which the Supreme Court held that the race of a stepparent could not be used as the basis for a custody determination, the Court has made clear that public biases cannot be used as the foundation for public policy. Although disregard for prevailing attitudes may make life more complicated or difficult, the Equal Protection clause bars consideration of prejudice or its effects when the government acts. Fear is not a legitimate basis for state action.

Although the Court narrowly upheld the constitutionality of state sodomy laws (*Bowers v. Hardwick*, 1986), most of the judicial opinions that subsequently have cited *Palmore* have involved attempts to discriminate against gay men, lesbians, or people with HIV infection (majority opinions: *Buttino v. Federal Bureau of Investigation*, 1992 [FBI agent fired because of his homosexuality]; *Citizens for Responsible Behavior v. Superior Court*, 1991 [initiative to repeal ordinance prohibiting discrimination on the basis of sexual orientation]; *Conkel v. Conkel*, 1987 [visitation by a bisexual father]; *Doe v. District of Columbia*, 1992 [HIV-positive individual denied employment as a firefighter]; *In re B & F Associates, Inc.*, 1985 [lease for a gay bar]; *M. A. B. v. R. B.*, 1986 [custody dispute involving a gay father]; *Pruitt v. Cheney*, 1992 [lesbian soldier]; concurring opinion: *Watkins v. U.S. Army*, 1989 [gay soldier]; dissenting opinions: *Bowers v. Hardwick*, 1986 [criminal charge of sodomy]; *Naragon v. Wharton*, 1984 [lesbian teaching assistant fired because of a relationship with a student]).[1]

Most courts have demanded that states and municipalities that seek to confirm private biases against homosexuals justify their action, and most have found that even a rational-basis test (the lowest level of scrutiny) cannot be met. In denying a ballot initiative to overturn an antidiscrimination

---

1. For other cases in which *Palmore* has been cited, see *City of Cleburne v. Cleburne Living Center*, 1985 (zoning ordinance prohibiting group home for people with mental retardation); *Michelle W. v. Ronald M.*, 1985 (interracial custody dispute), dissenting opinion; *State v. French*, 1990 (landlord discrimination against an unmarried couple), dissenting opinion; *State v. Shillcutt*, 1984 (racial slur by a juror), dissenting opinion.

ordinance, for example, a California appellate court described the initiative as having the "patent objective of fostering and furthering private discrimination" (*Citizens for Responsible Behavior v. Superior Court*, 1991, 2 Cal. Rptr. 2d at 21). The court added that "[a]ll that is lacking is a sack of stones for throwing" (2 Cal. Rptr. 2d at 30).

Perhaps no court has been as vociferous, though, in attacking unjustified discrimination on the basis of HIV infection as has the federal district court of Nebraska. The court held that a mental retardation agency's plan to require HIV-antibody testing of its staff violated the Equal Protection clause:

> The evidence, considered in its entirety, leads to the conclusion that the policy was prompted by concerns about the AIDS virus, formulated with little or erroneous medical knowledge, and is a constitutionally impermissible reaction to a devastating disease with no known cure. The risk of transmission of the disease from the staff to the clients at [the agency] is minuscule, trivial, extremely low, extraordinarily low, theoretical, and approaches zero. Such a risk does not justify the implementation of such a sweeping policy that ignores and violates the staff members' constitutional rights. (*Glover v. Eastern Nebraska Office of Retardation*, 1988, p. 251)

The Role of Science in Quelling Fear

Just as the Nebraska court alluded to medical knowledge, the tradition in public health law has been to show deference to the judgments of health care professionals. Operating on the principle of self-defense, courts have been willing to use medical judgments to justify substantial intrusion into the lives of people to protect the public health (see *Jacobson v. Massachusetts*, 1905, for the foundation case in this regard). In recent times, however, such opinions have been relied upon more to limit than to justify coercive and discriminatory action (see, e.g., *New York State Association for Retarded Children v. Carey*, 1979; *Whalen v. Roe*, 1977).

In the Supreme Court's most impassioned reliance on health care professionals' opinions (in that instance, an amicus curiae brief [advising the court on some legal matter] within the purview of the author of the brief by the American Medical Association), the Court held that Section 504 of the Rehabilitation Act of 1973 (1988) bars the use of fear as a basis for government-sanctioned discrimination:

By amending the definition of "handicapped individual" to include not only those who are actually physically impaired, but also those who are regarded as impaired and who, as a result, are substantially limited in a major life activity, Congress acknowledged that society's accumulated myths and fears about disability and disease are as handicapping as are the physical limitations that flow from actual impairment. . . . The Act is carefully structured to replace such reflexive reactions to actual or perceived handicaps with actions based on reasoned and medically sound judgments. . . . The fact that some persons who have contagious diseases may pose a serious health threat to others under certain circumstances does not justify excluding from the coverage of the Act all persons with actual or perceived contagious diseases. Such exclusion would mean that those accused of being contagious would never have the opportunity to have their condition evaluated in light of medical evidence and a determination made as to whether they were "otherwise qualified." Rather, they would be vulnerable to discrimination on the basis of mythology—precisely the type of injury Congress sought to prevent. (*School Board v. Arline*, 1987, pp. 284–285)

The significance of this statement in the present context is that health researchers bear a special responsibility to be "out front" in combating "mythology" that is used to rationalize discrimination. There is a duty not only to promote human welfare (for example, to develop the knowledge relevant to prevention and treatment of disease) but also to do so in a manner that alleviates unrealistic fear among many members of the public and sometimes the health professions themselves.

Melton described previously the most fundamental interest at stake: "The fact that an individual has a disease should not be cause in itself to treat him or her as a leper. (The irony of the analogy is intentional.) A debilitating, life-threatening illness creates its own kind of prison, but that fact should not diminish personhood. A weak body diminishes dignity only if society permits it to do so, and government [and researchers] should not collude in action that degrades any of its citizens" (Henggeler et al., 1992, p. 128).

The avoidance of such collusion requires affirmative efforts. Scientists who sit passively on the sideline not only will not have an impact in alleviating a great social and health crisis but also will often find that the political and social conflict is so great that they will be unable to do "pure" AIDS-related research.

At the beginning of this book, we noted the complexity of researchers' own interests—including their personal rewards—in AIDS research. In the end, we wish to commend those researchers who do their work diligently and thoughtfully with sensitivity to the interests of research participants. In that regard, we offer the comments of Don Des Jarlais, perhaps the most important researcher on AIDS among IV-drug users and a member of the National Commission on AIDS. Having been "burned" in political squabbles surrounding the Commission's work and vilified by some for efforts to experiment with needle exchanges, Des Jarlais's approach is philosophical but impassioned:

> Conducting research on controversial topics is seldom easy. The studies are usually technically difficult, and there are sensitive ethical and cultural problems to be addressed. Funding may be difficult to obtain; [for example,] to date, the federal government has refused to fund syringe exchange research and major surveys of sexual behavior. Researchers can expect bitter personal attacks even for proposing studies. They can also expect that, whatever their ultimate findings might be, the results will undergo distortion in both the political and media arenas. Nevertheless, datafree policymaking is likely to exacerbate rather than solve public health problems. Researchers with the requisite skills and opportunities who decide not to conduct research on important and controversial topics should be considered to have failed their ethical responsibilities to the persons who might have benefitted from the research. (Des Jarlais & Stepherson, 1991, p. 1394)

There is no greater antidote to unwarranted fear than knowledge. Researchers on AIDS have the opportunity to build a less acrimonious and fearful society, but to do so they must be thoughtful and willing to withstand critical views, and they must give due consideration to the experiences and beliefs of the affected communities.

As Morin observed in the Foreword to this volume, "the AIDS epidemic has taught us many lessons." To be sure, it has sharpened our acuity by bringing these issues into stark focus. But the issues are not germane exclusively to AIDS research. Research, as a means through which knowledge is acquired, is intended to improve the human condition. The AIDS pandemic has reminded us of this by providing us with a clear example of a human condition much in need of improvement.

Research must go on, within and during the AIDS crisis and beyond.

We must remain steadfastly committed to our goal of improving human-kind, however slowly and, at times, painfully. We must also be mindful of the fact that incremental benefits to all of us often accumulate only at the expense of incremental losses to some of us. Thus, we must strive to min-imize the losses and maximize the benefits so that the answer to the question "Was it worth it?" is, "Yes."

REFERENCES

Acquired Immune Deficiency Syndrome Research Confidentiality Act, *Cal. Health and Safety Code* §§ 119.30–199.40 (West 1990).

Additional Protections for Children Involved as Subjects in Research, 45 C.F.R. §§ 46.401–46.409 (1993).

Additional Protections Pertaining to Research, Development, and Related Activities Involving Fetuses, Pregnant Women, and Human in Vitro Fertilization, 45 C.F.R. §§ 46.201–46.211 (1992).

Adler, T. (1992a, February). Needle exchange helps, but isn't enough. *APA Monitor*, p. 34.

Adler, T. (1992b, February). Physicians can be helped not to fear HIV patients. *APA Monitor*, p. 11.

Adler, T. (1992c, April). Intervention is designed to boost HIV drug trials: High dropout rates, noncompliance issues tackled by psychologists in AZT study. *APA Monitor*, p. 22.

Alberts v. Devine, 479 N.E.2d 113 (1985), *cert.* denied, 474 U.S. 1013 (1986).

American Law Institute. (1965). *Restatement of torts* (2nd ed.). St. Paul, MN: Author.

American Medical Association, Council on Ethical and Judicial Affairs (1988, June). *Ethical issues involved in the growing AIDS crisis*. Washington, DC: Author.

American Psychological Association. (1992). Ethical principles of psychologists and code of conduct. *American Psychologist, 47*, 1597–1611.

American Sociological Association. (1982). *Code of ethics*. Washington, DC: Author.

Americans with Disabilities Act of 1990, 42 U.S.C. §§ 12101–12213 (Supp. III 1991).

Anderson, W. (1991). The New York needle trial: The politics of public health in the age of AIDS. *American Journal of Public Health, 81*, 1506–1517.

Andrews v. Eli Lilly & Co., 97 F.R.D. 494 (N.D. Ill. 1983), vacated *sub nom.* Deitchman v. E. R. Squibb & Sons, Inc, 740 F.2d 556 (1984).

Andrulonis v. United States, 924 F.2d 1210 (2d Cir. 1991) (Andrulonis v. United States I), *cert.* granted and rev'd *and* remanded *for reconsideration*, 112 S.Ct. 39 (1991), aff'd, 952 F.2d 652 (1991).

Angell, M. (1988). Ethical imperialism? Ethics in international collaborative clinical research. *New England Journal of Medicine, 319,* 1081–1083.

Annas, G. J., Glantz, L. H., & Katz, B. F. (1977). *Informed consent to human experimentation.* Cambridge, MA: Ballinger.

Anonymous. (1990). [Letter to the editor]. *New England Journal of Medicine, 322,* 1392.

Apicella v. McNeil Laboratories, Inc., 66 F.R.D. 78 (1975).

Application of R. J. Reynolds Tobacco Co., 518 N.Y.S. 2d 729 (N.Y. Sup. Ct. 1987).

Areen, J. (1992). Legal constraints on social research with children. In B. Stanley & J. E. Sieber (Eds.), *Social research on children and adolescents: Ethical issues* (pp. 7–28). Newbury Park, CA: Sage.

Arline v. School Board of Nassau County, 772 F.2d 759 (11th Cir. 1985), reh'g denied, 481 U.S. 1024 (1987); aff'd, School Bd. of Nassau County v. Arline, 480 U.S. 273 (1987).

Association of State and Territorial Health Officers. (1987). *Guide to public health practice: AIDS confidentiality and anti-discrimination principles: Interim report.* Washington, DC: Author.

Auerbach, D. M., Darrow, W. W., Jaffe, H. W., & Curran, J. W. (1984). Cluster of cases of the acquired immune deficiency syndrome: Patients linked by sexual contact. *American Journal of Medicine, 76,* 487–492.

Baker v. F & F Inc., 470 F.2d 778 (2d Cir. 1972), *cert.* denied, 411 U.S. 966 (1973).

Banks v. Bethlehem Steel Corp., 870 F.2d 1438 (9th Cir. 1989).

Barber, B., Lally, J., Makaruska, J., & Sullivan, R. D. (1973). *Research on human subjects; problems of social control in medical experimentation.* New York: Russell Sage Foundation.

Barefoot v. Estelle, 463 U.S. 880 (1983).

Barre-Sinoussi, F., Cherman, J. C., Ray, F., Nygeyre, M. T., Chamaret, S., Gruest, J., Dauget, C., Axler-Blin, C., Vezinet-Brun, F., Rouzioux, C., Rozenbaum, W., & Montagnier, L. (1983). Isolation of a T-lymphotropic retrovirus from a patient at risk for acquired immune deficiency syndrome (AIDS). *Science, 220,* 868–871.

Barry, M. (1988). Ethical considerations of human investigation in developing countries: The AIDS dilemma. *New England Journal of Medicine, 319,* 1083–1086.

Batchelor, W. F. (1988). AIDS 1988: The science and the limits of science. *American Psychologist, 43,* 853–858.

Bayer, R. (1989). *Private acts, social consequences: AIDS and the politics of public health.* New York: Free Press.

Bayer, R., Levine, C., & Murray, T. H. (1984). Guidelines for confidentiality in research on AIDS. *IRB: A Review of Human Subject Research, 6*(6), 1–7.

Bayer, R., Levine, C., & Wolf, S. M. (1986). HIV antibody screening: An ethical framework for evaluating proposed programs. *Journal of the American Medical Association, 256,* 1768–1774.

Becker, C. E., Cone, J. E., & Gerberding, J. (1989). Occupational infection with human immunodeficiency virus. *Annals of Internal Medicine, 110,* 653–666.

Becker, M. H., & Joseph, J. G. (1988). AIDS and behavioral change to reduce risk: A review. *American Journal of Public Health, 78,* 394–410.

Beecher, H. E. (1966). Ethics and clinical research. *New England Journal of Medicine, 274,* 1354–1360.

Belitsky, R., & Solomon, R. A. (1987). Doctors and patients: Responsibilities in a confidential relationship. In H. L. Dalton, S. Burris, & the Yale AIDS Project (Eds.), *AIDS and the law: A guide for the public* (pp. 201–209). New Haven, CT: Yale University Press.

Belle Bonfils Memorial Blood Center v. Denver District Court, 763 P.2d 1003 (1988).

Belmont report: Ethical principles and guidelines for research involving human subjects. (1979). Washington, DC: U.S. Department of Health, Education, and Welfare.

Bennett, C. L., Garfinkle, J. B., Greenfield, S., Draper, D., Rogers, W., Mathews, W. C., & Kanouse, D. (1989). The relation between hospital experience and in-hospital mortality for patients with AIDS-related PCP. *Journal of the American Medical Association, 261,* 2975–2979.

Bertrand, J. T., Makani, B., Hasig, S. E., Niwembo, K. L., Djunghu, B., Muanda, M., & Chirhamsolekwa, C. (1991). AIDS-related knowledge, sexual behavior, and condom use among men and women in Kinshasha, Zaire. *American Journal of Public Health, 81,* 53–58.

Blank v. Talley Indus., Inc., 54 F.R.D. 627 (S.D.N.Y. 1972).

Board of Trade of City of Chicago v. Commodity Futures Trading Commission, 627 F.2d 392 (D.C.Cir. 1980).

Boness, F. H., & Cordes, J. (1973). The researcher-subject relationship: The need for protection and a model statute. *Georgetown Law Journal, 62,* 243–272.

Boruch, R. F., & Cecil, J. S. (1979). *Assuring the confidentiality of social research data.* Philadelphia: University of Pennsylvania Press.

Bosk, C. L., & Frader, J. E. (1991). AIDS and its impact on medical work: The culture and politics of the shop floor. In D. Nelkin, D. P. Willis, & S. V. Parris (Eds.), *A disease of society: Cultural and institutional responses to AIDS* (pp. 150–171). Cambridge, England: Cambridge University Press.

Bower, R. T., & de Gasparis, P. (1978). *Ethics in social research: Protecting the interests of human subjects.* New York: Praeger.

Bowers v. Hardwick, 478 U.S. 186 (1986).

Brady v. Hopper, 751 F.2d 329 (10th Cir. 1983).

Brandt, A. M. (1988). AIDS in historical perspective: Four lessons from the history of sexually transmitted diseases. *American Journal of Public Health, 78,* 367–371.

Branzburg v. Hayes, 408 U.S. 665 (1972).

Breger, M. J. (1983). Randomized social experiments and the law. In R. F. Boruch & J. S. Cecil (Eds.), *Solutions to ethical and legal problems in social research* (pp. 97–144). New York: Academic Press.

Bridge, T. P. (1988a). AIDS and HIV CNS disease: A neuropsychiatric disorder. In T. P. Bridge, A. F. Mirsky, & F. K. Goodwin (Eds.), *Psychological, neuropsychiatric, and substance abuse aspects of AIDS* (pp. 1–13). New York: Raven.

Bridge, T. P. (1988b). Introduction. In T. P. Bridge, A. F. Mirsky, & F. K. Goodwin (Eds.), *Psychological, neuropsychiatric, and substance abuse aspects of AIDS* (pp. vii-ix). New York: Raven.

Brook, I. (1987). Approval of zidovudine (AZT) for acquired immunodeficiency syndrome: A challenge to the medical and pharmaceutical communities. *Journal of the American Medical Association, 258*(11), 1517.

Brown, B. P. (1983). Free press, privacy, and privilege: Protection of researcher-subject communications. *Georgetown Law Review, 17*, 1009–1048.

Buchanan v. American Motors Corp., 697 F.2d 151 (6th Cir. 1983).

Budiansky, S. (1983). Confidential matters. *Nature, 304,* 478.

Bulkley, J. (1981). Analysis of civil child protection statutes dealing with sexual abuse. In J. Bulkley (Ed.), *Child sexual abuse and the law* (pp. 81–88). Washington, DC: American Bar Association.

Buttino v. Federal Bureau of Investigation, 801 F.Supp 298 (1992).

Carl Zeiss Stiftung v. V. E. B. Carl Zeiss, 40 F.R.D. 318 (D.D.C. 1966), aff'd, V. E. B. Carl Zeiss, Jena, Steelmasters Inc. v. Clark, 384 F.2d 979 (1967).

Carter, W. (1978). *Some educational and political considerations in validating tests used as one criterion in the employment of public school teachers.* Paper presented at the meeting of the Evaluation Network, Aspen, CO.

Case, P., Merideth, G., Garcia, D., Tavera, H., Clark, G., & Wagner, T. (1992). Needle exchange: From civil disobedience to public policy. *Multicultural Inquiry and Research on AIDS, 4*(4), 1–3.

Celanese Corp. v. E. I. duPont de Nemours & Co., 58 F.R.D. 606 (D.Del. 1973).

Centers for Disease Control. (1981). Kaposi's sarcoma and *Pneumocystis* pneumonia among homosexual men: New York City and California. *Morbidity and Mortality Weekly Report, 30,* 305–308.

Centers for Disease Control. (1982). A cluster of Kaposi's sarcoma and *Pneumocystis carinii* pneumonia among homosexual male residents of Los Angeles and Orange Counties, California. *Morbidity and Mortality Weekly Report, 31,* 305–307.

Centers for Disease Control. (1985a). Recommendations for assisting in the prevention of perinatal transmission of human T-lymphotropic virus type III/lymphadenopathy-associated virus and acquired immunodeficiency syndrome. *Morbidity and Mortality Weekly Report, 34,* 721–732.

Centers for Disease Control. (1985b). Update: Acquired immunodeficiency syndrome: United States. *Morbidity and Mortality Weekly Report, 34,* 245–248.

Centers for Disease Control. (1988). Partner notification for preventing human immunodeficiency virus (HIV) infection. *Morbidity and Mortality Weekly Report, 37,* 393–404.

Check, J. V. P., & Malamuth, N. M. (1984). Can there be positive effects of participation in pornography experiments? *Journal of Sex Research, 20,* 14–31.

Chrysler Corp. v. Brown, 441 U.S. 281 (1979).

Ciba-Geigy v. Matthews, 428 F.Supp. 523 (S.D.N.Y. 1977).

Citizens for Responsible Behavior v. Superior Court, 1 Cal. App. 4th 1013, 2 Cal. Rptr. 648 (1991).

City of Cleburne, Texas v. Cleburne Living Center, 473 U.S.432 (1985).

Cleary, P. D., Barry, M. J., Mayer, K. H., Brandt, A. M., Gostin, L., & Fineberg, H. V. (1987). Compulsory premarital screening for the human immunodeficiency virus: Technical and public health considerations. *Journal of the American Medical Association, 258,* 1757–1762.

Cleary, P. D., Van Devanter, N., Rogers, T. F., Singer, E., Shipton-Levy, R., Steilen, M., Stuart, A., Avorn, J., & Pindyck, J. (1993). Depressive symptoms in blood donors notified of HIV infection. *American Journal of Public Health, 83,* 534–539.

Coates, T. J., Stall, R. D., Kegeles, S. M., Lo, B., Morin, S. B., & McKusick, L. (1988). AIDS antibody testing: Will it stop the AIDS epidemic? Will it help people infected with HIV? *American Psychologist, 43,* 859–864.

Cochran, S. D., & Mays, V. M. (1990). Sex, lies, and H.I.V. *The New England Journal of Medicine, 322,* 774–775.

Cohen, R. J. (1979). *Malpractice: A guide for mental health professionals.* New York: Free Press.

Cohen, S. I. (1988). Voodoo death, the stress response, and AIDS. In T. P. Bridge, A. F. Mirsky, & F. K. Goodwin (Eds.), *Psychological, neuropsychiatric, and substance abuse aspects of AIDS* (pp. 95–109). New York: Raven.

Collins, C. J. (1984). AIDS legal guide: Confidentiality. In A. R. Rubenfeld (Ed.), *AIDS legal guide: A professional resource on AIDS-related issues and discrimination* (pp. 16–21). New York: Lambda Legal Defense and Education Fund.

Colvard, R. (1967). Interaction and identification in reporting field research: A critical reconsideration of protective procedures. In G. Sjoberg (Ed.), *Ethics, politics and social research* (pp. 319–358). Cambridge, MA: Schenkman.

Committee for the Protection of Human Participants in Research. (1985, July). Ethical issues in psychological research on AIDS. *APA Monitor,* p. 26 (Reprinted in *IRB: A Review of Human Subjects Research,* 8(4), 8–10, 1986, and *Journal of Homosexuality, 13*(1), 93–101, 1986).

Committee for the Protection of Human Participants in Research, American Psychological Association. (1982). *Ethical principles in the conduct of research with human participants.* Washington, DC: American Psychological Association.

Communicable Disease Prevention and Control Act of 1987, *Tex. Health and Safety Code* § 81.001–81.009 (West 1992).

Community alert. (1993, Summer). *Psychology & AIDS Exchange,* p. 1.

Comprehensive Alcohol Abuse and Alcoholism Prevention, Treatment, and Rehabilitation Act Amendments of 1974, Pub. L. No. 93–282, 88 Stat. 127 (codified as amended in scattered sections of 42 U.S.C.).

Conkel v. Conkel, 31 Ohio App. 3d 169, 509 N.E.2d 983 (1987).

Controlled Substances Act, 21 U.S.C. §§ 801–904 (1988).

Cooper v. Florida, 539 So.2d 508 (Fla. App., 1989).

County of Westchester v. People, 122 A.D.2d 1 (N.Y. App. 1986).

Cruise, K. R., Jacobs, J. E., & Lyons, P. M., Jr. (1994). Definitions of physical abuse: A preliminary inquiry into children's perceptions. *Behavioral Sciences and the Law, 12,* 35–48.

Curran, W. J., Gostin, L. O., & Clark, M. E. (1986). *Acquired immunodeficiency syndrome: Legal and regulatory policy* (Contract No. 282–86–0052). Washington, DC: National Technical Information Service.

Curran, W. J., Jaffe, H. W., Hardy, A. M., Morgan, W. M., Selik, R. M., & Dondero, T. J. (1988). Epidemiology of HIV infection and AIDS in the United States. *Science, 239* (4840), 610–617.

Currie v. United States, 644 F.Supp 1074 (M.D.N.C. 1986), aff'd, Currie v. U.S., 836 F.2d 209 (1987).

Curtis, J. L., Crummey, F. C., Baker, S. N., Foster, R. E., Khanyile, C. S., & Wilkins, R. (1989). HIV screening and counseling for intravenous drug abuse patients: Staff and patient attitudes. *Journal of the American Medical Association, 261,* 258–262.

Cutler J. C., & Arnold, R. C. (1988). Venereal disease control by health departments in the past: Lessons for the present. *American Journal of Public Health, 78,* 372–376.

Davis v. Rodman, 227 S.W. 612 (Ark. 1921).

Deitchman v. E. R. Squibb & Sons, Inc., 740 F.2d 556 (7th Cir. 1984).

DeKraai, M. B., & Sales, B. D. (1984). Confidential communications of psychotherapists. *Psychotherapy, 21,* 293–318.

Department of Air Force v. Rose, 425 U.S. 352 (1976).

Department of Health, Education, and Welfare (1973, November 16). Protection of human subjects: Policies and procedures. *Federal Register, 38* (221 Part II), 31737–31749.

Des Jarlais, D. C., & Friedman, S. R. (1988). The psychology of preventing AIDS among intravenous drug users: A social learning conceptualization. *American Psychologist, 43,* 865–870.

Des Jarlais, D. C., & Stepherson, B. (1991). History, ethics, and politics in AIDS prevention research. *American Journal of Public Health, 81,* 1393–1394.

Diaz, T., Buehler, J. W., Castro, K. G., & Ward, J. W. (1993). AIDS trends among Hispanics in the United States. *American Journal of Public Health, 83,* 504–509.

Dickens, B. M. (1988). Legal limits of AIDS confidentiality. *Journal of the American Medical Association, 259,* 3449–3551.

Doe v. District of Columbia, 796 F.Supp. 559 (D.D.C. 1992).

Doe v. Prime Health/Kansas City, Inc. No. 88-C-5149, slip op. at 11 (Dist. Ct. Johnson County, Kan., Oct. 18, 1988).

Dow Chemical Co. v. Allen, 672 F.2d 1262 (7th Cir. 1982).

Eckler, A. R. (1972). *The bureau of the census.* New York: Praeger.

Edgar, H., & Rothman, D. J. (1991). New rules for new drugs: The challenge of AIDS to the regulatory process. In D. Nelkin, D. P. Willis, & S. V. Parris (Eds.), *A disease of society: Cultural and institutional responses to AIDS* (pp. 84–115). Cambridge, England: Cambridge University Press.

EEOC v. University of Notre Dame Du Lac, 715 F.2d 331 (7th Cir. 1983).

Eglin Federal Credit Union v. Cantor, Fitzgerald Sec. Corp., 91 F.R.D. 414 (N.D. Ga. 1981).

Elifson, K. W., Boles, J., Posey, E., Sweat, M., Darrow, W., & Elsea, W. (1993).

Male transvestite prostitutes and HIV risk. *American Journal of Public Health, 83*, 260–262.

Elwork, A., Sales, B. D., & Alfini, J. J. (1982). *Making jury instructions understandable*. Charlottesville, VA: Michie.

Emerson, T. I. (1970). *The system of freedom of expression*. New York: Random House.

Employee Retirement Income Security Act of 1974, 29 U.S.C. §§ 1001–1461 (1988).

Excerpts from Report by AIDS Panel Chairman. (1988, June 3). *New York Times*, p. 16.

Farnsworth v. Procter & Gamble Co., 758 F.2d 1545 (11th Cir. 1985).

Federal researcher predicts HIV vaccine will be ready to test within three years. (1992, July 24). *AIDS Policy and Law, 7*(14), pp. 4–5.

Fellner, C. H., & Marshall, J. R. (1970). Kidney donors: The myth of informed consent. *American Journal of Psychiatry, 126*, 1245–1251.

Fischl, M. A., Richman, D. D., Grieco, M. H., Gottleib, M. S., Volberding, P. A., Laskin, O. L., Leedom, J. M., Groopman, J. E., Mildvan, D., Schooley, R. T., Jackson, G. G., Durack, D. T., King, D., and AZT Collaborative Group. (1987). The efficacy of azidothymidine (AZT) in the treatment of patients with AIDS and AIDS-related complex: A double-blind, placebo-controlled trial. *New England Journal of Medicine, 317*, 185–191.

Flaherty, D. H. (1978). Final report of the Bellagio Conference on Privacy, Confidentiality, and the use of government microdata for research and statistical purposes. *Statistical Reporter, 78*(8), 274–279.

Florida Stat. Anno. § 827.07(2)(D)(1) (1976).

Food and Drug Administration. (1989a, January). IRB information sheet: Significant differences in HHS and FDA regulations for IRBs and informed consent (FDA IRB Information Sheets, pp. 85–87). Washington, DC: Department of Health and Human Services.

Food and Drug Administration. (1989b, February). IRB information sheet: Answers to frequently asked questions (FDA IRB Information Sheets, pp. 23–34). Washington, DC: Department of Health and Human Services.

Food and Drug Administration. (1989c, May). Clinical investigator information sheet: Informed consent and the clinical investigator (FDA Clinical Investigator Information Sheets, pp. 10–17). Washington, DC: Department of Health and Human Services.

Forsham v. Califano, 587 F.2d 1128 (D.C. Cir. 1978), aff'd *sub nom.* Forsham v. Harris 445 U.S. 169 (1980).

Forsham v. Harris, 445 U.S. 169 (1980).

Fortin, A. J. (1991). Ethics, culture, and medical power: AIDS research in the Third World. *AIDS and Public Policy Journal, 6*, 15–24.

Fox, R., Odaka, N. J., Brookmeyer, R., & Polk, B. F. (1987). Effect of HIV antibody disclosure on subsequent sexual activity in homosexual men. *AIDS, 1*, 241–246.

Freedom of Information Act, 5 U.S.C. § 552 (1988).

Freeman v. Seligson, 405 F.2d 1326 (D.C. Cir. 1968).

Freiberg, P. (1994). More at table to spend AIDS monies. *APA Monitor, 25*(2), 32–33.

Friedman, S. R. (1992). Drug injectors and HIV: New issues arise, yet many old ones remain unresolved. *AIDS and Public Policy Journal, 7,* 137–140.

F.T.C. v. Shaffner, 626 F.2d 32 (7th Cir. 1980).

F.T.C. v. Texaco, Inc., 555 F.2d 862 (D.C.Cir. 1977).

Fulero, S. M. (1988). *Tarasoff*: 10 years later. *Professional Psychology: Research and Practice, 19*(2), 184–190.

Fullilove, R. E., Fullilove, M. T., Bowser, B. P., & Gross, S. A. (1990). Risk of sexually transmitted disease among black adolescent crack users in Oakland and San Francisco, California. *Journal of the American Medical Association, 263,* 851–855 (© 1990, American Medical Association).

Gallo, R. C., Salhuddin, S. A., Popovic, M., Shearer, G. M., Kaplan, M., Haynes, B. F., Palker, T. J., Redfield, R., Oleske, J., Safai, B., White, G., Foster, P., & Markham, P. D. (1984). Frequent detection and isolation of cytopathic retroviruses (HTLV-III) from patients with AIDS and at risk for AIDS. *Science, 224,* 500–503.

Gammill v. United States, 727 F.2d 950 (10th Cir. 1984).

General Accounting Office. (1989). AIDS education: Issues affecting counseling and testing programs (GAO Publication No. HRD-89-39). Washington, DC: U.S. Government Printing Office. (ERIC Document Reproduction Service No. ED 306 483).

General Motors Corporation v. Director of National Institute for Occupational Safety and Health, 636 F.2d 163 (6th Cir. 1980).

Georgia Power Co. v. EEOC, 295 F.Supp. 950 (N.D.Ga. 1968), aff'd, 412 F.2d 462 (1969).

Getman v. NLRB, 450 F.2d 670 (D.C.Cir. 1971).

Girardi, J. A., Keese, R. M., Traver, L. B., & Cooksey, D. R. (1988). Featured debate: Psychotherapist responsibility in notifying individuals at risk for exposure to HIV. *Journal of Sex Research, 25,* 1–27.

Glaser, R., & Kiecolt-Glaser, J. K. (1988). Stress-associated immune suppression and acquired immune deficiency syndrome (AIDS). In T. P. Bridge, A. F. Mirsky, & F. K. Goodwin (Eds.), *Psychological, neuropsychiatric, and substance abuse aspects of AIDS* (pp. 203–215). New York: Raven.

Glover v. Eastern Nebraska Office of Retardation, 686 F. Supp. 243 (D.Neb.1988), aff'd, 867 F.2d 461 (8th Cir. 1989), *cert.* denied, 492 U.S. 916 *and* 493 U.S. 932 (1989).

Goodgame, R. W. (1990). AIDS in Uganda: Clinical and social features. *New England Journal of Medicine, 323,* 383–389.

Gordis, L., & Gold, E. (1980). Privacy, confidentiality, and the use of the medical records in research. *Science, 207,* 153–156.

Gostin, L. O. (1989). Public health strategies for confronting AIDS: Legislative and regulatory policy in the United States. *Journal of the American Medical Association, 261,* 1621–1630.

Gostin, L. O. (1990a). The AIDS Litigation Project: A national review of court and human rights commission decisions. Part I. The social impact of AIDS. *Journal of the American Medical Association, 263,* 1961–1970.

Gostin, L. O. (1990b). The AIDS Litigation Project: A national review of court and human rights commission decisions. Part II. Discrimination. *Journal of the American Medical Association, 263,* 2086–2093.

Gostin, L. O., & Curran, W. J. (1987). Legal control measures for AIDS: Reporting requirements, surveillance, quarantine, and regulation of public meeting places. *American Journal of Public Health, 77,* 214–218.

Gostin, L. O., Curran, W. J., & Clark, M. E. (1987). The case against compulsory casefinding in controlling AIDS-testing, screening and reporting. *American Journal of Law and Medicine, 12,* 7–53.

Gottlieb, M. S., Schroff, R., Shanker, H. M., Weisman, J. D., Phan, P. T., Wolf, R. A., & Saxon, A. S. (1981). *Pneumocystis carinii* pneumonia and mucosal candidiasis in previously healthy homosexual men: Evidence for a new acquired cellular immunodeficiency. *New England Journal of Medicine, 305,* 1425–1431.

Grattan v. People, 65 N.Y.2d 243, 491 N.Y.S.2d 125 (1985).

Gray, B. H. (1975). *Human subjects in medical experimentation: A sociological study of the conduct and regulation of clinical research.* New York: Wiley.

Gray, J. N. (1989). Pediatric AIDS research: Legal, ethical and policy influences. In J. M. Seibert & R. A. Olson (Eds.), *Children, adolescents and AIDS* (pp. 179–227). Lincoln: University of Nebraska Press.

Gray, J. N., & Melton, G. B. (1985). The law and ethics of psychosocial research on AIDS. *Nebraska Law Review, 64,* 637–688.

Green, S. T., Goldberg, D. J., Nathwani, D., Christie, P. R., & Thomson, A. (1990). Intercourse during menstruation among prostitutes. *Journal of the American Medical Association, 264,* 333.

Greenstein, R. L. (1984). Federal contractors and grantees: What are your First Amendment rights? *Jurimetrics Journal, 24,* 197–209.

Grisso, T. (1992). Minors' assent to behavioral research without parent permission. In B. Stanley & J. E. Sieber (Eds.), *Social research on children and adolescents: Ethical issues* (pp. 109–127). Newbury Park, CA: Sage.

Grisso, T. (in press). Voluntary consent to research participation in the institutional context. In B. H. Stanley, J. E. Sieber, & G. B. Melton (Eds.), *Research ethics: A psychological approach.* Lincoln: University of Nebraska Press.

Griswold v. Connecticut, 381 U.S. 479 (1965).

Grund, J.-P. C., Kaplan, C. D., & Adriaans, N. F. P. (1991). Needle sharing in the Netherlands: An ethnographic analysis. *American Journal of Public Health, 81,* 1602–1607.

Grundner, T. M. (1978). Two formulas for determining the readability of subject consent forms. *American Psychologist, 33,* 773–775.

Gurevitz, H. (1977). *Tarasoff*: Protective privilege versus public peril. *American Journal of Psychiatry, 134,* 289–292.

H. Kessler & Co. v. EEOC, 53 F.R.D. 330 (N.D.Ga. 1971), *cert.* denied, 412 U.S. 939 (1973), aff'd, 468 F.2d 25 (1972), modified, 472 F.2d 1147 (1973).

Hafemeister, T. L., & Amirshahi, A. J. (1992). Civil commitment for drug dependency: The judicial response. *Loyola of L. A. Law Review, 26*(1), 39–104.

Hamilton, D. P. (1991). Hints emerge from the Gallo probe. *Science, 253,* 728–729.

Hardy, L. M. (Ed.). (1991). *HIV screening of pregnant women and newborns.* Washington, DC: National Academy Press.

Hasenei v. United States, 541 F.Supp. 999 (D. Md. 1982).

Hawaii Psychiatric Society v. Ariyoshi, 481 F. Supp. 1028 (D. Hawaii 1979).

Health Omnibus Programs Extension of 1988, Pub. L. No. 100–607, 102 Stat. 3048 (codified as amended in scattered sections of 42 U.S.C.).

Hein, K. (1991). Fighting AIDS in adolescents. *Issues in Science and Technology, 7*(3), 67–72.

Henderson, D. K., Fahey, B. J., Willy, M., Schmitt, J. M., Carey, K., Koziol, D. E., Lane, H. C., Fedio, J., & Saah, A. J. (1990). Risk for occupational transmission of human immunodeficiency virus type 1 (HIV-1) associated with clinical exposures: A prospective evaluation. *Annals of Internal Medicine, 113,* 740–746.

Henggeler, S. W., Melton, G. B., & Rodrigue, J. (1992). *Pediatric and adolescent AIDS: Research findings from the social sciences.* Newbury Park, CA: Sage.

Herek, G. M., & Capitanio, J. P. (in press). Conspiracies, contagion, and compassion: Trust and public reactions to AIDS. *AIDS Education and Prevention.*

Herek, G. M., & Glunt, E. K. (1988). An epidemic of stigma: Public reactions to AIDS. *American Psychologist, 43,* 886–891.

Herek, G. M., Kimmel, D. C., Amaro, H., & Melton, G. B. (1991). Avoiding heterosexist bias in psychological research. *American Psychologist, 46,* 957–963.

Herman, R. (1987, October 9). Pasteur's leader in AIDS research. *International Herald Tribune,* p. 20.

Hershey, N. (1976). Putting teeth into the public health reporting laws. *American Journal of Public Health, 66,* 399–400.

Hilts, P. J. (1993, November 13). U.S. drops misconduct case against an AIDS researcher. *New York Times,* p. 1.

Hirschel, B., Lazzarin, A., Chopard, P., Opravil, M., Furrer, H. J., Ruttiman, S., Vernazza, P., Chave, J.-P., Ancarani, F., Gabriel, V., Heald, A., King, R., Malinveri, R., Martin, J.-L., Mermillod, B., Nicod, L., Simoni, L., Vivirito, M. C., Zerboni, R., & Swiss Group for Clinical Studies on AIDS. (1991). A controlled study of inhaled pentamidine for primary prevention of *Pneumocystis carinii* pneumonia. *New England Journal of Medicine, 324,* 1079–1083.

Hofmann v. Blackman, 241 So.2d 752 (Fla. App. 1970).

Holder, A. R. (1993). Research records and subpoenas: A continuing issue. *IRB: A Review of Human Subjects Research, 15*(1), 6–7.

Hooker, T. (1992). Getting to the point: HIV, drug abuse and syringe exchange in the United States. *State Legislative Report, 17*(14).

Huszti, H. C., & Chitwood, D. D. (1989). Prevention of pediatric and adolescent AIDS. In J. M. Seibert & R. A. Olson (Eds.), *Children, adolescents, & AIDS* (pp. 147–177). Lincoln: University of Nebraska Press.

Illinois passes controversial AIDS bills. (1988, June 10). *San Francisco Sentinel,* p. 13.

In re B & F Associates, Inc., 55 B.R. 19 (Bankr. D.D.C. 1985).

In re Dinnan, 661 F.2d 426 (5th Cir. 1981).

In re District 27 Community School Board v. Board of Education of the City of New York, 502 N.Y.S. 2d 325 (N.Y. Sup. Ct., Queens County 1986).

In re Grand Jury Subpoena Dated January 4, 1984, 750 F.2d 223 (2d Cir. 1984).

In re Grand Jury Subpoena Dated Jan. 4, 1984, 583 F.Supp. 991 (E.D.N.Y. 1984), rev'd., 750 F.2d 223 (2d Cir. 1984).

In re January 1976 Grand Jury, 534 F.2d 719 (7th Cir. 1976).

In re Penn Central Commercial Paper Litigation, 61 F.R.D. 453 (S.D.N.Y. 1973).

In re Snyder, 115 R.F.D. 211 (D.Ariz. 1987).

Institut Pasteur v. United States, 814 F.2d 624 (Fed. Cir. 1987).

Institute of Medicine. (1991). *The AIDS research program of the National Institutes of Health.* Washington, DC: National Academy Press.

Jablonski ex rel. Pahls v. United States, 712 F.2d 391 (9th Cir. 1983).

Jacobson v. Massachusetts, 197 U.S. 11 (1905).

Jenny, C., Hooton, T., Bowers, A., Copass, M. K., Krieger, J. N., Hillier, S. L., Kiviat, N., Corey, L., Stamm, W. E., & Holmes, K. K. (1990). Sexually transmitted diseases in victims of rape. *New England Journal of Medicine, 322,* 713–716.

Jew Ho v. Williamson, 103 F. 10 (N.D. Cal. 1900).

John Citizen v. City Health Project (In G. J. Wood & A. Philipson, AIDS, testing, and privacy: An analysis of case histories. (1987). *AIDS and Public Policy Journal, 2*(3), 1–25).

Jonsen, A. R. (1989). Foreword. In E. T. Juengst & Barbara A. Koenig (Eds.), *The meaning of AIDS: Implications for medical science, clinical practice, and public health policy* (pp. xi–xiii). New York: Praeger.

Joseph, J. G., Montgomery, C., & Kirscht, J. (1987). Perceived risk of AIDS: Assessing the behavioral and psychological consequences in a cohort of gay men. *Journal of Applied Psychology, 17,* 231–250.

Jurek v. Texas, 428 U.S. 262 (1976).

Juvenile Justice Standards Project. (1977). *Standards relating to abuse and neglect.* Cambridge, MA: Ballinger.

Kaplan, E. H. (1988). Crisis? A brief critique of Masters, Johnson and Kolodny. *Journal of Sex Research, 25,* 317–322.

Katz, J. (1972). *Experimentation with human beings.* New York: Sage.

Katz, J. (1978). Informed consent: A fairy tale? Law's vision. *University of Pittsburgh Law Review, 27,* 137–154.

Katz, J. (1984). *The silent world of doctor and patient.* New York: Free Press.

Katz v. United States, 389 U.S. 347 (1967).

Keeling, R. P. (1986). Introduction. In R. P. Keeling (Ed.), *AIDS on the college campus: ACHA special report* (pp. vii–xii). Rockville, MD: American College Health Association.

Keith-Spiegel, P. (1983). Children and consent to participate in research. In G. B. Melton, G. P. Koocher, & M. J. Saks (Eds.), *Children's competence to consent* (pp. 179–211). New York: Plenum.

Keith-Spiegel, P., & Koocher, G. P. (1985). *Ethics in psychology: professional standards and cases.* New York: Random House.

Kelly, J. A., St. Lawrence, J. S., Hood, H. V., Smith, S., Jr., & Cook, D. J. (1987a).

Medical students' attitudes toward AIDS. *Journal of Medical Education, 62,* 549–556.

Kelly, J. A., St. Lawrence, J. S., Hood, H. V., Smith, S., Jr., & Cook, D. J. (1987b). Stigmatization of AIDS patients by physicians. *American Journal of Public Health, 77,* 789–791.

Kennedy v. Connecticut Department of Public Safety, 115 F.R.D. 497 (D.Conn. 1987).

Kershaw, D. N., & Small, J. C. (1972). Data, confidentiality and privacy: Lessons from the New Jersey negative income tax experiment. *Public Policy, 20,* 257–280.

Khabbaz, R. F., Darrow, W. W., Hartley, T. M., Witte, J., Cohen, J. B., French, J., Gill, P. S., Potterat, J., Sikes, R. K., Reich, R., Kaplan, J. E., & Lairmore, M. D. (1990). Seroprevalence and risk factors for HTLV-I/II infection among female prostitutes in the United States. *Journal of the American Medical Association, 263,* 60–64.

Kidder, L., & Brickman, P. (1971). When directness is the better part of valor: Effects of normative and informational pressure on direct and indirect attitude tests. *Journal of Personality and Social Psychology, 18,* 238–246.

Kiecolt-Glaser, J. K., & Glaser, R. (1988). Major life changes, chronic stress, and immunity. In T. P. Bridge, A. F. Mirsky, & F. K. Goodwin (Eds.), *Psychological, neuropsychiatric, and substance abuse aspects of AIDS* (pp. 217–224). New York: Raven.

Klovdahl, A. S. (1985). Social networks and the spread of infectious diseases: The AIDS example. *Social Science and Medicine, 21,* 1203–1216.

Kolata, G. (1993, March 7). Targeting urged in attack on AIDS: A neighborhood focus could halt spread, some argue. *New York Times,* pp. 1, 16.

Koocher, G. P., & O'Malley, J. E. (1981). *The Damocles syndrome.* New York: McGraw-Hill.

Korematsu v. United States, 323 U.S. 214 (1944).

Krauskopf, J. M., & Krauskopf, C. J. (1965). Torts and psychologists. *Journal of Counseling Psychology, 12,* 227–237.

Kreiss, J. K., Koech, D., Plummer, F. A., Holmes, K. K., Lightfoote, M., Piot, P., Ronald, A. R., Ndinya-Achola, M. B., D'Costa, L. J., Roberts, P., Ngugi, E. N., & Quinn, T. C. (1986). AIDS virus infection in Nairobi prostitutes: Spread of the epidemic to East Africa. *New England Journal of Medicine, 314,* 414–418.

Lampshire v. Procter & Gamble, 94 F.R.D. 58 (N.D. Ga. 1982).

Levering v. Commonwealth, 132 Ky. 666 (1909).

Levine, C. (1991). Women and HIV/AIDS research: The barriers to equity. *IRB: A Review of Human Subjects Research, 13*(1/2), 18–22.

Levine, C., Dubler, N. N., & Levine, R. J. (1991). Building a new consensus: Ethical principles and policies for clinical research on HIV/AIDS. *IRB: A Review of Human Subjects Research, 13*(1/2), 1–17.

Lewis, C. E., Freeman, H. E., & Corey, C. E. (1987). AIDS-related competence of California's primary care physicians. *American Journal of Public Health, 77,* 795–799.

Lidz, C. W. (1977). *The voluntariness of the voluntary patient: The weather report model of informed consent.* Paper presented at the VI World Congress of Psychiatry, Honolulu, HI.

Lidz, C. W., Meisel, A., Zerubavel, E., Carter, M., Sestak, R., & Roth, L. (1984). *Informed consent: A study of decisionmaking in psychiatry.* New York: Guilford Press.

Lidz, C. W., & Roth, L. H. (1983). The signed form: Informed consent? In R. F. Boruch & J. S. Cecil (Eds.), *Solutions to ethical and legal problems in social research* (pp. 145–157). New York: Academic Press.

Lipari v. Sears, Roebuck & Co., 497 F.Supp. 185 (D. Neb. 1980).

Lora v. Board of Education, 74 F.R.D. 565 (E.D.N.Y. 1977).

Lundgren v. Fultz, 354 N.W.2d 25 (Minn. 1984).

Lyter, D. W., Valdiserri, R. O., Kingsley, L. A., Amoroso, W. P., & Rinaldo, C. R., Jr. (1987). The HIV antibody test: Why gay and bisexual men want or do not want to know their results. *Public Health Reports, 102,* 468–474.

M. A. B. v. R. B., 134 Misc.2d 317, 510 N.Y.S.2d 960 (1986).

MacDonald, N. E., Wells, G. A., Fisher, W. A., Warren, W. K., King, M. A., Doherty, J. A., & Bowie, W. R. (1990). High risk STD/HIV behavior among college students. *Journal of the American Medical Association, 263,* 3155–3159.

Mann, J. (1988, January). *Global AIDS: Epidemiology, impact, projections, and the global strategy.* Invited address to the International Meeting of Health Ministers, London, England.

Marks, R. (1992). Magical thinking. *Focus: A Guide to AIDS Research and Counseling, 8,* 2.

Marwick, C. (1983). Confidentiality issues may cloud epidemiologic studies of AIDS. *Journal of the American Medical Association, 250,* 1945–1946.

Marwick, C. (1987). AZT (zidovudine) just a step away from FDA approval for AIDS therapy. *Journal of the American Medical Association, 257,* 1281–1282.

Marzuk, P. M., Tierney, H., Tarfidd, K., Gross, E. M., Morgan, E. B., Hsu, M. A., & Mann, J. G. (1988). Increased risk of suicide in persons with AIDS. *Journal of the American Medical Association, 259,* 1332–1333.

Masters, W. H., Johnson, V. E., & Kolodny, R. C. (1988). *Crisis: Heterosexual behavior in the age of AIDS.* New York: Grove Press.

Matherne, J. G. (1984). Forced disclosure of academic research. *Vanderbilt Law Review, 37,* 585–620.

Matthews, G. W., & Neslund, V. S. (1986). The initial impact of AIDS on public health law in the United States—1986. *Journal of the American Medical Association, 257,* 344–352.

McCusick, L. (1990). The story of the valiant attempt of the 1990 International AIDS Conference to make itself relevant to the community—with a review of program elements. *Multicultural Inquiry and Research on AIDS, 4*(2), 3–4.

McCusker, J., Stoddard, A. M., Mayer, K. H., Zapka, J., Morrison, C., & Saltzman, S. P. (1988). Effects of HIV antibody test knowledge on subsequent sexual behaviors in a cohort of homosexually active men. *American Journal of Public Health, 78,* 462–467.

McGann v. H. & H. Music Co., 946 F.2d 401 (5th Cir. 1991), modified sub *nom.* Greenberg v. H. & H. Music Co., 112 S.Ct. 1556 (1992), *cert.* denied 113 S.Ct. 482 (1992).

McKillip, J. (1991). The effect of mandatory premarital HIV testing on marriage: The case of Illinois. *American Journal of Public Health, 81*, 650–653.

McKinney's Consolidated Laws of New York Anno., 45 Public Health Law Art. 23 (I) § 2306 (1992).

McKinney's Consolidated Laws of New York Anno., 45 Public Health Law Art. 23 (F) § 2782 (1993).

McLean, P. D. (1980). The effect of informed consent on the acceptance of random treatment assignment in a clinical population. *Behavior Therapy, 11*, 129–133.

Meisel, A. (1977). The expansion of liability for medical accident: From negligence to strict liability by way of informed consent. *Nebraska Law Review, 56*, 51–152.

Melton, G. B. (1983). Minors and privacy: Are legal and psychological concepts compatible? *Nebraska Law Review, 62*, 455–493.

Melton, G. B. (1988). Ethical and legal issues in AIDS-related practice. *American Psychologist, 43*, 941–947.

Melton, G. B. (1989). Ethical and legal issues in research and intervention. *Journal of Adolescent Health Care, 10*, 36S–44S.

Melton, G. B (1990). Certificates of confidentiality under the Public Health Service Act: Strong protection but not enough. *Violence and Victims, 5*, 67–71.

Melton, G. B. (1991a). Ethical judgments amid uncertainty: Dilemmas in the AIDS epidemic. *Counseling Psychologist, 19*, 561–565.

Melton, G. B. (1991b). Respecting boundaries: Minors, privacy, and behavioral research. In B. Stanley & H. E. Sieber (Eds.), *Social research on children and adolescents: Ethical issues* (pp. 65–84). Lincoln: University of Nebraska Press.

Melton, G. B. (1992). The law is a good thing (psychology is, too): Human rights in psychological jurisprudence. *Law and Human Behavior, 16*, 381–398.

Melton, G. B., & Gray, J. N. (1988). Ethical dilemmas in AIDS research: Individual privacy and public health. *American Psychologist, 43*, 60–64.

Melton, G. B., Koocher, G. P., & Saks, M. J. (Eds.). (1983). *Children's competence to consent.* New York: Plenum.

Melton, G. B., Levine, R. J., Koocher, G. P., Rosenthal, R., & Thompson, W. C. (1988). Community consultation in socially sensitive research: Lessons from clinical trials of treatments for AIDS. *American Psychologist, 43*, 573–581.

Melton, G. B., Petrila, J., Poythress, N. C., & Slobogin, C. (1987). *Psychological evaluations for the courts: A handbook for mental health professionals and lawyers.* New York: Guilford.

Melton, G. B., & Stanley, B. H. (in press). Research involving special populations. In B. H. Stanley, H. E. Sieber, & G. B. Melton (Eds.), *Research ethics: A psychological approach.* Lincoln: University of Nebraska Press.

Merigan, T. C. (1989). A personal view of efforts in treatment of human immunodeficiency virus infection in 1988. *Journal of Infectious Diseases, 159*, 390–399.

Merriken v. Cressman, 364 F.Supp. 913 (E.D. Pa. 1973).

Michaels, D., & Levine, C. (1992). Estimates of the number of motherless youth orphaned by AIDS in the United States. *Journal of the American Medical Association, 268,* 3456–3461.

Michelle W. v. Ronald W., 703 P.2d 88, (Cal. 1985), appeal dismissed, 474 U.S. 1043 (1986).

Miller, H. G., Turner, C. G., & Moses, L. E. (Eds.). (1990). *AIDS: The second decade.* Washington, DC: National Academy Press.

Mills, M., Wofsy, C. B., & Mills, J. (1986). The acquired immunodeficiency syndrome: Infection control and public health law. *The New England Journal of Medicine, 314,* 931–936.

Minnesota v. Andring, 342 N.W.2d 128 (Minn. 1984).

Monahan, J. (1993, March). Limiting therapist exposure to *Tarasoff* Liability: Guidelines for risk containment. *American Psychologist, 48,* 242–250.

Morin, S. F. (1987, August 6). [Testimony on behalf of the American Psychological Association before the House Health and the Environment Subcommittee on the subject of AIDS legislation.]

Morris, R. A., Sales, B. D., & Berman, J. J. (1981). Research and the freedom of information act. *American Psychologist, 36,* 819–826.

Moss, A. R. (1989). Coercive and voluntary policies in the AIDS epidemic. In E. T. Juengst & B. A. Koenig (Eds.), *The meaning of AIDS: Implications for medical science, clinical practice, and public health policy* (pp. 174–183). New York: Praeger.

Naragon v. Wharton, 737 F.2d 1403 (5th Cir. 1984).

National Commission for the Protection of Human Subjects in Biomedical and Behavioral Research. (1977). *Report and recommendations: Research involving children* (DHEW publication (OS) 77–0004). Washington DC: U.S. Department of Health, Education, and Welfare.

National Commission for the Protection of Human Subjects in Biomedical and Behavioral Research. (1979). *The Belmont report: Ethical principles and guidelines for the protection of human subjects of research* (DHEW publication (OS) 78–0012). Washington, DC: U.S. Department of Health, Education, and Welfare.

National Institute for Occupational Safety and Health. (1989). Guidelines for prevention of transmission of human immunodeficiency virus and hepatitis B virus to health-care and public-safety workers. *Morbidity and Mortality Weekly Report, 38*(S-6).

Navia, B. A., Jordan, B. D., & Price, R. W. (1986). The AIDS dementia complex: I.Clinical features. *Annals of Neurology, 19,* 517–524.

Nebraska Mental Health Commitment Act of 1976, *Nebraska Revised Statutes* §§ 83–1001 to 1078 (1992).

Nelkin, D. (1984). *Science as intellectual property: Who controls scientific research?* New York: Macmillan.

Nelson, L. J. (1989). Law, ethics, and advance directives regarding the medical care of AIDS patients. In E. T. Juengst & B. A. Koenig (Eds.), *The meaning of AIDS: Implications for medical science, clinical practice, and public health policy* (pp. 94–100). New York: Praeger.

New York Family Court Act, § 1012 (1983), 45 *New York Public Health Law* 2782(4)(9)(3) (McKinney 1993).

New York State Association for Retarded Children v. Carey, 612 F.2d 644 (2d Cir. 1979).

New York Testing Confidentiality Act of 1988, *New York Public Health Law* 2785 (1993).

Nichols, E. (1991). *Expanding access to investigational therapies for HIV infection and AIDS.* Washington, DC: National Academy Press.

NIH agency begins study of AZT for effectiveness in pregnancy. (1991). *AIDS Policy and Law,* 6(10), pp. 2–3.

1993 Revised classification system for HIV infection and expanded surveillance case definition for AIDS among adolescents and adults. (1993). *Journal of the American Medical Association,* 269(6), 729–730.

Nolan, K. (1990). AIDS and pediatrics research. *Evaluation Review,* 14, 464–481.

Norman, C. (1985). Patent dispute divides AIDS researchers. *Science, 230,* 640–643.

Novick, A. (1984). At risk for AIDS: Confidentiality in research and surveillance, *IRB: A Review of Human Subjects Research,* 6(6), 10–11.

Novick, A. (1990a). May a human subject waive the right to be treated as a human subject? *AIDS and Public Policy Journal, 5,* 45–48.

Novick, A. (1990b). Noncompliance in clinical trials: II. Primary care physicians. *AIDS and Public Policy Journal, 5,* 142–144.

Nuremburg Code (1947). Reprinted in *Science, 1964, 143,* 553.

Office for Protection from Research Risks, National Institutes of Health. (1984). *Guidance for Institutional Review Boards for AIDS Studies.* Bethesda, MD: Author.

Office of Technology Assessment. (1985). *Review of the public health service's responses to AIDS: A technical memorandum.* Washington, DC: Author.

Ohio-Sealy Mattress Mfg. Co. v. Sealy, Inc., 90 F.R.D. 45 (N.D.Ill. 1981).

Oklahoma Press Publishing Co. v. Walling, 327 U.S. 186 (1946).

Oleske, J., Minnefor, A., Cooper, R., Thomas, K., Cruz, A., Ahdieh, H., Guerrero, I., Joshi, V. V., & Desposito, F. (1983). Immune deficiency syndrome in children. *Journal of the American Medical Association,* 249, 2345–2349.

Osmond, D. (1992). Ethical and legal issues of vaccine clinical trials. *Focus: A Guide to AIDS Research and Counseling,* 8(1), 1–4.

Owens v. Storehouse, 773 F.Supp. 416 (N.D. Ga. 1991), aff'd, 984 F.2d 394 (1993).

Palca, J. (1991). Popovic blasts accusers, demands report be withdrawn. *Science, 253,* 729–731.

Palmore v. Sidoti, 466 U.S. 429 (1984).

Panem, S. (1984). AIDS, public policy, and biomedical research. *Chest,* 85, 416–422.

Pape, J. W., Verdier, R.-I., & Johnson, W. D., Jr. (1989). Treatment and prophylaxis of *Isospora belli* infection in patients with the acquired immunodeficiency syndrome. *New England Journal of Medicine,* 320, 1044–1047.

Parmet, W. E. (1981). Public Health Protection and the Privacy of Medical Records, *Harvard Civil Rights-Civil Liberties Law Review, 16,* 265–304.

Partner notification: State and local health officials urge adoption of contact tracing programs. (1988, November 30). *AIDS Policy and Law,* pp. 1, 12.

Peck v. Counseling Service of Addison County, Inc., 499 A.2d 422 (Vt. 1985).

Price, M. E. (1989a, August 7). Searching for a new paradigm. *National Law Journal,* pp. 13–14, 16–17.

Price, M. E. (1989b). *Shattered mirrors: Our search for identity and community in the AIDS era.* Cambridge, MA: Harvard University Press.

Privacy Act of 1974, 5 U.S.C. § 552a (1988).

Protection of Human Subjects, 7 C.F.R. §§ 1c.101–.124 (1993) [Agriculture].

Protection of Human Subjects, 10 C.F.R. §§ 745.101–.124 (1993) [Energy].

Protection of Human Subjects, 14 C.F.R. §§ 1230.101–.124 (1993) [National Aeronautics and Space Administration].

Protection of Human Subjects, 15 C.F.R. §§ 27.101–.124 (1993) [Commerce].

Protection of Human Subjects, 16 C.F.R. §§ 1028.101–.124 (1993) [Consumer Product Safety Commission].

Protection of Human Subjects, 22 C.F.R. §§ 225.101–.124 (1993) [Agency for International Development].

Protection of Human Subjects, 24 C.F.R. §§ 60.101–.124 (1993) [Housing and Urban Development].

Protection of Human Subjects, 28 C.F.R. §§ 46.101–.124 (1993) [Justice].

Protection of Human Subjects, 32 C.F.R. §§ 219.101–.124 (1993) [Defense].

Protection of Human Subjects, 34 C.F.R. §§ 97.101–.124 (1992) [Education].

Protection of Human Subjects, 38 C.F.R. §§ 16.101–.124 (1993) [Veterans Affairs].

Protection of Human Subjects, 40 C.F.R. §§ 26.101–.124 (1992) [Environmental Protection Agency].

Protection of Human Subjects, 45 C.F.R. §§ 46.101–.124 (1992) [Health and Human Services].

Protection of Human Subjects, 45 C.F.R. §§ 690.101–.124 (1992) [National Science Foundation].

Protection of Human Subjects, 49 C.F.R. §§ 11.101–.124 (1992) [Transportation].

Pruitt v. Cheney, 963 F.2d 1160 (9th Cir. 1992), *cert.* denied, 113 S.Ct. 655.

Public Health Service Act, 42 U.S.C. §§ 201 to 300aaa-3 (1988).

Rasmussen v. South Florida Blood Service, Inc., 500 So.2d 533 (Fla. 1987).

Rehabilitation Act of 1973, 29 U.S.C. §§ 701–701, 720–724, 730–732, 740–741, 750, 760–764, 770–776, 780–787, & 790–794 (1988).

Richards of Rockford Publishing Co. v. Pacific Gas & Elec., 71 F.R.D. 388 (N.D. Cal. 1976).

Richwald, G. A., Morisky, D. E., Kyle, G. R., Kristal, A. R., Gerber, M. M., & Friedland, J. M. (1988). Sexual activities in bathhouses in Los Angeles County: Implications for AIDS prevention education. *Journal of Sex Research, 25,* 169–180.

Robiner, W. N., Parker, S. A., Ohnsorg, T. J., & Strike, B. (1993). HIV/AIDS training and continuing education for psychologists. *Professional Psychology: Research and Practice, 24,* 35–42.

Robinson v. Magovern, 83 F.R.D. 79 (W.D. Pa. 1979).

Roth, L. H., Lidz, C. W., Meisel, A., Soloff, P. H., Kaufman, K., Spiker, D. G., & Foster, F. G. (1982). Competency to decide about treatment or research: An overview of some empirical data. *International Journal of Law and Psychiatry, 5,* 29–50.

Roth, L. H., Meisel, A., & Lidz, C. W. (1977). Tests of competency to consent to treatment. *American Journal of Psychiatry, 134*(3), 279–284.

Rubinstein, E.(1991). The Gallo factor: Questions remain. *Science, 253,* 732.

Ruebhausen, O. M., & Brim, O. E. (1966). Privacy and behavioral research. *American Psychologist, 21,* 423–444.

Rural Housing Alliance v. U.S. Department of Agriculture, 498 F.2d 73 (D.C. Cir. 1974).

Schachter v. Whalen, 581 F.2d 35 (2d Cir. 1978).

Schlorer, J. (1975). Identification and retrieval of personal records from a statistical data bank. *Methods of Information in Medicine, 14,* 7–13.

Schoenbaum, E. E., Hartel, D., Selwyn, P. A., Klein, R. S., Davenny, K., Rogers, M., Feiner, C., & Friedland, G. (1989). Risk factors for human immunodeficiency virus infection in intravenous drug users. *New England Journal of Medicine, 321,* 874–879.

Schoenbaum, E. E., & Webber, M. P. (1993). The underrecognition of HIV infection in women in an inner-city emergency room. *American Journal of Public Health, 83*(3), 363–368.

School Board of Nassau County v. Arline, 480 U.S. 273 (1987).

Seibert, J. M., & Olson, R. A. (eds.). (1989). Children, adolescents, and AIDS. Lincoln: University of Nebraska Press.

Sherman, R. (1991, October 14). Criminal prosecutions on AIDS growing. *National Law Journal,* pp. 3, 38.

Shilts, R. (1987). *And the band played on: People, politics, and the AIDS epidemic.* New York: St. Martin's Press.

Siegel, D. D. (1992). Federal subpoena practice under the new rule 45 of the federal rules of civil procedure. *Federal rules decisions, 139,* 197–239.

Sims v. Central Intelligence Agency, 642 F.2d 562 (D.C. Cir. 1980).

Singer, E. (1978). Informed consent: Consequences for response rate and response quality in social surveys. *American Sociological Review, 3,* 144–162.

Singer, E. (1983). Informed consent procedures in surveys: Some reasons for minimal effects on responses. In R. F. Boruch & J. S. Cecil (Eds.), *Solutions to ethical and legal problems in social research* (pp. 183–212). New York: Academic Press.

Small, M. A. (1988, March). *Factors in privacy expectations.* Paper presented at the meeting of the American Psychology-Law Society, Miami.

Stall, R. D., Coates, T. J., & Hoff, C. (1988). Behavioral risk reduction for HIV infection among gay and bisexual men: A review of results from the United States. *American Psychologist, 43,* 878–885.

Stanley, B. (1987). Informed consent in treatment and research. In I. B. Weiner & A. K. Hess (Eds.), *Handbook of forensic psychology* (pp. 63–85). New York: Wiley.

State and local health officials urge adoption of contact tracing programs. (1988, December 14). *AIDS Policy and Law, 3*(23), pp. 1, 12.

State v. French, 460 N.W.2d 2 (Minn. 1990).

State v. Shillcutt, 350 N.W.2d 686 (Wis. 1984).

State-of-the-Art Conference on AZT Therapy for Early HIV Infection, National Institute of Allergy & Infectious Diseases. (1990). Recommendations for zidovudine: Early infection. *Journal of the American Medical Association, 263*, 1606, 1609.

Steinbrook, R., Lo, B., Moulton, J., Saika, G., Hollander, H., & Volberding, P. A. (1986). Preferences of homosexual men with AIDS for life-sustaining treatment. *New England Journal of Medicine, 314*, 457–460.

Sterling v. Bloom, 723 P.2d 755 (Idaho 1986).

Stryker, J. (1989). IV drug use and AIDS: Public policy and dirty needles. *Journal of Health Politics, Policy, and Law, 14*, 719–740.

Subcommittee on Disclosure-Avoidance Techniques (Committee on Federal Statistical Methodology). (1978). *Report on statistical disclosure and disclosure-avoidance techniques.* Washington, DC: U.S. Department of Commerce, Federal Statistical Policy and Standards.

Susser, M. (1993). Emancipate CDC. *American Journal of Public Health, 83*, 491–492.

Sweezy v. New Hampshire, 354 U.S. 234 (1957).

Tapp, J. L., & Melton, G. B. (1983). Preparing children for decision making: Implications of legal socialization research. In G. B. Melton, G. P. Koocher, & M. J. Saks (Eds.), *Children's competence to consent* (pp. 215–233). New York: Plenum.

Tarantola, D., & Mann, J. (1993, Spring). Coming to terms with the AIDS pandemic. *Issues in Science and Technology*, pp. 41–48.

Tarasoff v. Regents of the University of California (Tarasoff I), 529 P.2d 533 (Cal. 1974).

Tarasoff v. Regents of the University of California (Tarasoff II), 551 P.2d 334 (Cal. 1976).

Tavoulareas v. Piro, 93 F.R.D. 24 (D.D.C. 1981).

Taylor, R. (1993a, March). Live SIV vaccines get new respect. *Journal of NIH Research*, pp. 31–32.

Taylor, R. (1993b, February). Sex surveys help map AIDS risk. *Journal of NIH Research*, pp. 31–32.

Thomas, S. B., & Quinn, S. C. (1991). The Tuskegee syphilis study, 1932 to 1972: Implications for HIV education and AIDS risk education programs in the Black community. *American Journal of Public Health, 81*, 1498–1504.

Thurman, S. D. (1973). *The right of access to information from the government.* New York: Oceana.

Trammel v. U.S., 445 U.S. 40 (1980).

Turner, A. G. (1982). What subjects of survey research believe about confidentiality. In J. E. Sieber (Ed.), *The ethics of social research: Surveys and experiments* (pp. 151–163). New York: Springer-Verlag.

Turner, C. F., Miller, H. G., & Moses, L. E. (Eds.). (1989). *AIDS: Sexual behavior and intravenous drug use.* Washington, DC: National Academy Press.

United States v. Brandt, 1948 (reprinted in 1–2 Trials of War Criminals Before the Nuremburg Military Tribunals).

United States v. Doe, 460 F.2d 328 (1st Cir. 1972).

United States v. IBM, 83 F.R.D. 97 (S.D.N.Y. 1975).

United States v. Nixon, 418 U.S. 688 (1974).

United States v. Westinghouse Electric Corporation, 638 F.2d 570 (3d Cir. 1980).

Update: Reducing HIV transmission in intravenous-drug users not in drug treatment: United States. (1990). *Morbidity and Mortality Weekly Report, 39,* 529, 535–538.

Valdiserri, R. O. (1987). Epidemics in perspective. *Journal of Medical Humanities and Bioethics, 8,* 95–100.

Valdiserri, R. O., Tama, G. M., & Ho, M. (1988). The role of community advisory committees in clinical trials of anti-HIV agents. *IRB: A Review of Human Subjects Research, 10*(4), 5–7.

Valleroy, L. A. (1990, Autumn). Pediatric AIDS and HIV infection in the United States: Recommendations for research, policy, and programs. *Society for Research in Child Development Social Policy Report,* pp. 1–12.

Varmus, H. E. (1989). Naming the AIDS virus. In E. T. Juengst & B. A. Koenig (Eds.), *The meaning of AIDS: Implications for medical science, clinical practice, and public health policy* (pp. 3–11). New York: Praeger.

Vernon's Texas Codes Ann., Code of Criminal Procedure, Art. 21.31 (1992a).

Vernon's Texas Codes Ann., 2(D) Health and Safety Code 81(A) § 81.003–81.106 (1992b).

Volberding, P. A., Lagakos, S. W., Koch, M. A., Pettinelli, C., Myers, M. W., Booth, D. K., Balfour, H. H., Jr., Reichman, R. D., Bartlett, J. A., Hirsch, M. S., Murphy, R. L., Hardy, W. D., Soeiro, R., Fischl, M. A., Bartlett, J. G., Merigan, T. C., Hyslop, N. E., Richman, D. D., Valentine, F. T., Corey, L., & AIDS Clinical Trial Group of the National Institute of Allergy & Infectious Diseases. (1990). Zidovudine in asymptomatic human immunodeficiency virus infection: A controlled trial in persons with fewer than 500 CD4-positive cells per cubic millimeter. *New England Journal of Medicine, 322,* 941–949.

von Bulow v. von Bulow, 811 F.2d 136 (2d Cir. 1987), *cert.* denied, 481 U.S. 1015 (1987).

Washington v. Harper, 494 U.S. 210 (1990).

Washington Research Project v. Department of Health, Education, and Welfare, 504 F.2d 238 (D.C. Cir. 1974).

Watkins v. U.S. Army, 875 F.2d 699 (9th Cir. 1989).

Weithorn, L. A. (1983). Involving children in decisions affecting their own welfare: Guidelines for professionals. In G. B. Melton, G. P. Koocher, & M. J. Saks (Eds.), *Children's competence to consent* (pp. 235–260). New York: Plenum.

Westinghouse Elec. Corp. v. City of Burlington, 351 F.2d 762 (D.C. Cir. 1965).

Whalen v. Roe, 429 U.S. 589 (1977).

White, K., Kando, J., Park, T., Waternaux, C., & Brown, W. A. (1992). Side effects and the "blindability" of clinical drug trials. *American Journal of Psychiatry, 149*, 1730–1731.

Wigmore, J. H. (1961). *Evidence in trials at common law, Vol. 8*, Sec. 2285. Boston, MA: Little, Brown and Co.

Wilkerson, I. (1988, July 1). American Medical Association urges breach of privacy to warn potential AIDS victims. *New York Times*, p. 1.

Windom, R. E. (1986, September 19). [Statement to the press on the results of the clinical trial of AZT for treatment of people with AIDS]. Washington, DC: U.S. Department of Health and Human Services.

Windom, R. E. (1988, May 9). *Policy on informing those tested about HIV infection*. Washington, DC: Public Health Service.

Winslade, W. J., & Ross, J. W. (1985). Privacy, confidentiality and autonomy in psychotherapy. *Nebraska Law Review, 64*, 578–636.

Wood, G. J., & Philipson, A. (1987). AIDS, testing, and privacy: An analysis of case histories. *AIDS and Public Policy Journal, 2*, 21–25.

Woods v. White, 689 F. Supp. 874 (W.D. Wis. 1988), aff'd, 899 F.2d 17 (7th Cir. 1990).

Wright v. Jeep Corporation, 547 F.Supp. 871 (E.D. Mich., 1982).

Wykoff, R. F., Heath, C. W., Hollis, S. L., Leonard, S. T., Quiller, C. B., Jones, J. L., Artzrouni, M., & Parker, R. L. (1988). Contact tracing to identify human immunodeficiency virus infection in a rural community. *Journal of the American Medical Association, 259*, 3563–3566.

Wyoming Statutes Annotated, § 14-3-202(ii)(A) (1977).

Youngstrom, N. (1992, April). AIDS studies on IV drug users needed. *APA Monitor*, p. 31.

INDEX